100 BEST

Yoga & Pilates

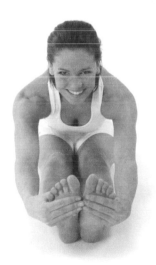

This edition published by Parragon Books Ltd in 2014
and distributed by

Parragon Inc.
440 Park Avenue South, 13th Floor
New York, NY 10016
www.parragon.com

Copyright © Parragon Books Ltd 2014

Designed by Stone Castle Graphics Limited
Additional Design Work by Talking Design
Compiled by Gillian Haslam

© Getty Images: pages 9, 11, 14, 15, 19ar, 21, 71, 97, 105 and 147
© Shutterstock.com: Yuri Arcurs 87; Phil Date 29, 51l Yellowj 13

ISBN 978-1-4723-6431-9

Printed in China

Picture acknowledgements
The publisher would like to thank the following for the permission to
reproduce copyright material on the front cover:
Woman sitting in yoga pose © Dimitri Otis / Getty Images (bottom
left)
Woman in yoga stretch © Mirko Iannace / Getty Images (top middle)
Woman practicing Pilates mat exercise, side view © Angela Coppola
/ Getty Images (bottom middle)
Instructor assisting woman with yoga position © Michael Goldman
/ Getty Images (bottom right)
Woman doing yoga © Robin Lewine / Getty Images (middle left)

Note:
As a precautionary measure, the publishers advise that anyone
intending to follow the exercise programs outlined in this book
should first consult a qualified practitioner or therapist.

100 BEST

Yoga & Pilates

The ultimate step-by-step exercises
for strength, flexibility, and control

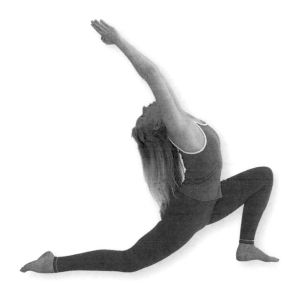

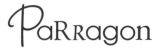

Bath · New York · Cologne · Melbourne · Delhi
Hong Kong · Shenzhen · Singapore · Amsterdam

CONTENTS

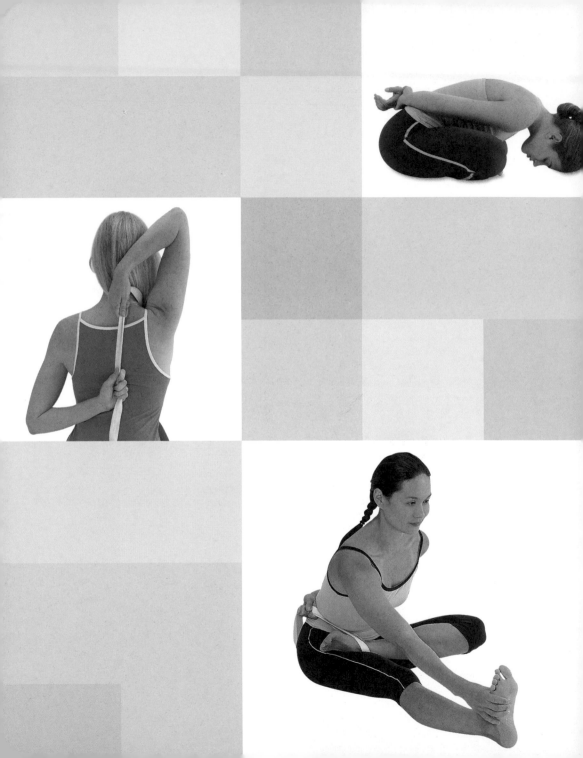

YOGA

INTRODUCTION

After their first yoga class, people often report that they've slept better and feel taller. Yoga has helped people lose weight, overcome fears, conquer habits like smoking, and develop better concentration, all of which help their performance in daily tasks. Others feel improved self-awareness, a deeper sense of well-being, developed compassion, enhanced relationships, greater self-acceptance, and a sensation of being at peace.

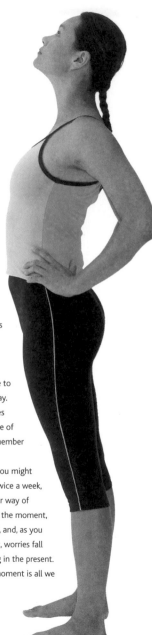

As we nudge our physical boundaries with yoga postures, we become fully focused on body, breath, and mind. We become absorbed in being in the present moment. It's a break from our usual mind status; it refreshes us. Yoga practice helps us move from distress to de-stress, from dis-ease to ease, from passion to compassion.

Contrary to what many believe, yoga is not a set of exercises or a meditation technique. It is actually a state of mind. The state of yoga is when the mind is still. The turnings of thoughts have ceased and there are no distractions. Over the last 2,000 years, other practices were developed that helped the body and mind become receptive to the experience of stillness. Of these practices, asana (physical postures) is the practice most commonly equated with yoga in the West. Stillness fosters awareness. Hatha yoga includes physical exercises that seek to relax and still the body; breath work to focus the mind; relaxation to quieten the body and mind; chanting to arouse and then calm the emotions; and meditation to center the spirit.

The word yoga originates from the Sanskrit word *yuj*. Yuj may be translated as "to center one's thoughts" or "to meditate deeply," both of which involve the slowing of the movements of the mind. From yuj also come "to unite" and "connect," which imply a reintegration, a bringing back into balance. It is often said that yoga means "union," because it harmonizes body, breath, mind, and spirit. But, paradoxically, yoga also seeks to disunite. The spirit, considered pure and eternal, separates from the physical body, and its purity is regained. Lastly, from the root *yuj* comes "to yoke." Yoking, or harnessing one's energies, connotes effort, and hatha yoga certainly requires this. The codes of moral conduct, physical exercises, breathing practices, concentration, and meditation all require effort, and all contribute to the goal

of self-realization. Keeping a healthy discipline makes life feel better. Sometimes you begin your practice feeling unfocused, lethargic, anxious, or tight in your body. Yet after absorbing yourself in your practice, you feel warm, loose, relaxed, calm, and perhaps more connected to a force greater than yourself.

Being off balance doesn't feel good—it's difficult to relate to others in a relaxed, authentic way. Fear fades and tranquillity arrives when you relax back into a sense of wholeness. It's when you re-remember who you are.

When you practice yoga, you might spend 30 minutes on the mat twice a week, or you might expand it into your way of life. When you are right there in the moment, there is nothing to work toward, and, as you mentally sink into that moment, worries fall away. Yoga lets us practice being in the present. The reality is that the present moment is all we really possess.

Right: *Yoga harmonizes body, breath, mind, and spirit.*

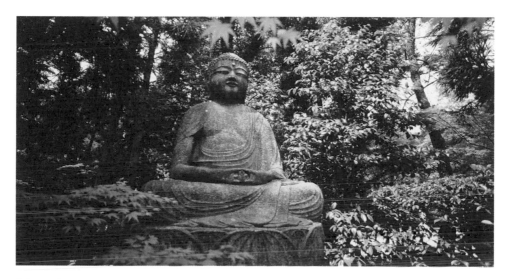

THE ASANAS

Watching my cats wake up is a lesson in itself. They reach forward and stretch back just like the yoga pose of Downward-Facing Dog. Then they round their backs while arching up (which we call Cat Pose) and yawn. Slow stretching is glorious It feels good and the body likes it. Your body wants to move and was designed for it. It feels better to be loose and free than to be all bound up, tense, and contracted.

A yoga "asana" is a posture where you are externally still, yet internally alive. To take part in asana practice is to use your body as the doorway through which to experience and remember the truth about who you are. By holding an asana we can integrate the body, breath, and mind.

One of the most common mental blocks for a beginner is the belief that they are not flexible enough for yoga. Advanced practitioners make the action look effortless. Many of the photos in this chapter are of teachers who have many years of asana practice. Mostly, the fullest forms of the asanas are shown. This is meant to inspire you, not discourage you!

As long as your alignment is not harming your body, it is not important whether or not your pose looks graceful. What matters is that you find the teaching point for that pose. It may be that, because of your body's individuality, you need to change the posture to fit you, rather than overriding your body's needs by forcing it to conform to an "ideal" shape. More than poise in the posture, it is the breath that should be graceful.

According to the Yoga-Sutra, the first codification of yoga, which dates back about 2,000 years, an asana must have the qualities of alertness and relaxation. It is perfected when no effort is necessary, hence relaxation is possible. Even if you feel like you have the flexibility of a block of wood, keep in mind the concept of "abhyasa," or "repeated effort." With repeated effort you cease to have to try.

Asanas help balance the body. They distribute strength and flexibility evenly between left and right, top and bottom, front and back. They develop strength in weaker areas of the body, and softness in tighter spots. Through freeing the outer body, asanas build and control the "prana"—the vital force—in the inner body. On an energetic level, polarity therapists believe the joints in the body can be weaker areas, and yoga postures mobilize and vitalize the joints.

Asanas focus the mind and are a way of coming back to the self. Like your body finding its center of gravity in a given position, finding just where your center is in your life is helpful. Asanas teach you that moving away from your center only creates internal conflict. Becoming more still, and therefore more aware, with yoga practice helps you notice when you are moving away from your center so you have the chance to bring yourself back.

Above: The ancient texts tell us that the state of yoga can be reached through dedication and practice.

THE BREATH

Your breath will bring your yoga alive. When you are consciously breathing, your practice can never be mechanical. Good breathing is reassuring, soothing, and healing. It will bring intuition to your postures. Remember that even in the seemingly stationary poses, when your body might be still on the outside, it is never stagnant. While there is breath awareness, there will be a feeling of cleansing, lightness, new energy, and mental clarity. If you forget your "breath" then come back to an exercise where the breath and movement are clearly linked so that you feel the flow. Holding the breath dulls the flow of feeling. If your breath freezes, ease the intensity of your posture, let the rhythm into the belly and chest once more, and catch the wave of the breath when it comes.

The breath is a mirror for your mind. Breath and mind are intrinsically connected. Any alteration in one will affect the other. The mind can multiply in ways that the breath cannot. As the breath is the slower-moving of the two, choosing to focus on it during asana practice will help to calm the churnings of thought. Awareness of the breath will draw your mind to the present moment. Evenness in your breath will be reflected in your mind. The breath is your monitor of how you are doing in the pose. When the breath flows steadily, your asana comes closer to being perfected.

Your natural breath can't be created by willpower alone. You can breathe freely only through releasing and undoing. The natural breath unshrinks and unkinks us and teaches us that sometimes the most subtle methods are the most profound. Come back to the breath often throughout the day and check how you are breathing.

Breathe in and out through the nose so that the air is filtered and warmed. To bring constancy to your breath, practice yoga asanas with a steady breath. In general, inhale on opening or unfolding the body, when performing rising or lengthening movements, when twisting the upper back, and when bending backward. Exhale when releasing, closing the body, moving downward, twisting the lower back, lowering the arms or legs, and when bending forward or sideways. These are general rules, but do experiment to intuit what feels right for your body. Try

a practice moving only on the exhalation, for example. The more slowly you move, the more easily awareness will come. In flowing postures, experiment with taking three or five breaths to complete a single movement. Remind yourself that it's irrelevant whether you can touch your toes or not. If you can breathe, you can practice yoga.

STAYING PRESENT

When you stay mentally present in a pose, awareness deepens. There are two types of asanas: conscious and unconscious. In a conscious position, the quality of the asana moves from that of body conditioner to become a psychospiritual exercise. When you are absorbed in the subtle sensations of the body, your mind is not permitted to dance away. Your mind will naturally run to the part of your body where the feelings are intense, but try to spread your awareness simultaneously and evenly over your body. From observing your hamstring in a forward bend, radiate your awareness to the whole leg, then keep radiating it until it touches the entire body.

If you spend one minute in a posture, observe, sense, visualize, and refine. Seek that still point, the epicenter of consciousness. Over the duration of your practice, these "one minutes" join together to create a unit of time during which you have been perfectly present. These blocks of time are healing and refreshing.

DOING AND UNDOING

Fully engaging a muscle will bring the mind right to that area. All-over awareness is excellent practice for concentration and being in the now. With the muscles engaged, the mind is engaged, and this is why yoga asanas have transformative power.

According to the Yoga-Sutra, an asana needs to be steady and comfortable. The stretching of yoga aims to expand, not strain. Strain blocks your ability to listen to what the body has to tell you. Go to the deepest you can, then hold it a little bit more. Non-harming is one of the precepts of yoga philosophy, and this certainly includes your treatment of your body. Overworking

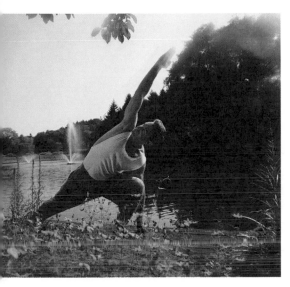

slow rhythmic movement may help. Flow in and out of the pose several times, before finally holding the pose. As you release the air from your lungs, release the tension in the body. Don't force; simply yield with each exhalation to extend farther. Let tension move out of your body and into the atmosphere.

ANCHORING AND RADIATING

With yoga, as in life, we need a base from which to move. When we are stable and grounded, directional movement can be focused. While one part of your body is well-grounded, another part can rise. When you anchor yourself securely, it makes the exercise more of a challenge. Often, less flexible people have a better yoga practice than those who are very flexible. Stiffer-bodied people know intuitively about anchoring and working from their base. People who are naturally flexible have to learn how to anchor themselves. Having a point from which to extend yourself is physiologically a bit like using weights in a gym. As you engage your muscles, there is a point from which to work.

Consider where your anchor is in each pose. The floor acts as your base when standing. As you take your arms overhead, extend and radiate upward from floor to fingertips. When you sit to bend forward, ground down through the sitting bones. When you lie prone to backbend, press down through the pubic bone and radiate out from the lower abdomen. When you sit to twist right, anchor the left buttock well down. In Shoulderstand, let the shoulders and elbows be heavy so the rest of the body can float lightly upward. When you hold your arms horizontal and stretch them apart, radiate your energy along the arms and reach outward, so that it feels like it is not just your muscular power holding them in place, but your mental energy stretching them away.

Our center of gravity lies 2 in (5 cm) below the navel. Learn to move from this center. This core acts as an anchor from which to extend. Then the movement from the center to the extremities feels integrated, and ripples of energy flow from our center to the rest of the body. Link them with the breath, the extension outward and the gentle rebounding flow back. Practice extending yourself without losing yourself.

your body is neglecting to take care, a form of misuse. Coax and persuade but don't force.

Some days it feels hard to pull yourself up out of your armchair. Other days you spring up effortlessly. When you engage the mind in the posture, you give strength to the posture. With strength comes a lovely feeling of lightness, too. It's like changing from a heavy, old car to a new one with power steering. When you have energy, strength, and lightness, it's much more pleasurable to move your body around.

On first meeting a posture, it might feel that it requires 100 percent effort to hold it. It can be hard to imagine being able to find any release in the pose at all. As you practice and become more comfortable with the pose, the effort required slowly reduces. With time and dedication, the proportion of doing to undoing will slide. The asana will feel more comfortable and more rewarding. Freedom comes into the pose.

We are accustomed to the concept of using effort to get somewhere. Letting go in order to achieve something might seem strange. Counter the effort of doing with plenty of undoing. Do more by doing less. If you are standing, enjoy the relief in surrendering your weight down through the soles of the feet. If you are sitting, sink down through the sitting bones. If you are balancing on your hands, soften the skin on the palms and release downward. This downward energy rebounds upward to be used in your posture. If the release won't come in a posture,

Above left and opposite: Yoga positions bring strength to weak areas of the body.

BANDHAS

A bandha involves the contraction of certain muscles to unlock the pranic vital energy so it can be directed upward. Bandhas may be used in conjunction with pranayama or asana practice to encourage the flow of the vital force and preserve it.

The bandhas are very useful during asana practice. They work with the organs, and the nervous and endocrine systems. They can improve disorders of the reproductive and urinary systems, sexual dysfunction, and back problems, and are helpful in the alleviation of problems experienced after childbirth.

The mulabandha is located at the perineum—the area between the anus and the genitals, and about 1 in (2.5 cm) in toward the core of the body. For women, it is also linked to the cervix. Uddhyanabandha is located in the core of the body just below the navel.

To practice with mulabandha and uddhyanabandha, sit erect. On your next inhalation, draw in the lower abdomen—the part just above the pubic bone and below the navel. As you do this, the perineum will lift slightly and a gentle mulabandha holding will be activated. Move between drawing in on the inhalation and letting go on the exhalation, so you get a sense of the lifting sensation in the pelvis.

When you are not used to isolating the mulabandha area, the surrounding muscles seem to want to tense up in sympathy. You might find your buttocks, thighs, and anus tightening, or that you are unconsciously holding your breath. In time, you will be able to more actively draw up the perineum without tensing other muscles.

The bandhas respond to different parts of the breath—while drawing in the lower abdomen is easiest on the inhalation, you might notice that actively drawing up the perineum feels easiest on an exhalation. Practice this while sitting, then incorporate it into forward bends and standing poses. Eventually, bring it into the other poses, too.

Above: During your practice you will experience strong sensations.

DISCOMFORT AND PAIN

During your practice you will feel intense sensations. The sensations you get from a strong stretch are not necessarily bad. You might feel discomfort, which is a "good hurt," or pain, a "negative hurt." Discomfort is resistance of the body or mind. When exploring new territory, mental and physical unease will inevitably arise.

Pain is more acute than discomfort. Discomfort, when caused by working strongly, is a positive feeling. With pain, there will be nothing pleasant about the soreness. Pain in a pose means you have overshot your limit by moving too quickly, or that you are improperly aligned. Pain is counterproductive, as the body will instinctively tense and move away from it. Pain in the muscles or joints could lead to injury, so never ignore it. Come out of the pose and examine your alignment or check with a teacher.

A high strain will force your attention away, while, if you are underworking your body, the mind will become lethargic. Optimum strain, working just at your edge, will engage your mind. When your body experiences a healthy amount of tension, you can move internally and tune in to the quietness. Remember that yoga seeks to remove pain and suffering, not increase it.

YOUR EDGE

Your edge is the point at which the strong challenge comes into the pose and where you feel you have reached a new frontier. During practice, aim to push back your edge in a slow, respectful way. Listen to your body's feedback, not only immediately after practice but over the following days. Each pose has many edges; each one is an opportunity to grow. As you approach your first edge, hold the position with a steady breath. Stay focused on that place in your body. Exhalation will help soften and prepare the body to move beyond it. Wait for your body to let you in. Should that inner cue come, proceed respectfully, with full attention. Then you have found a new edge. Likewise, it is good to be adventurous but this does not mean you should be aggressive.

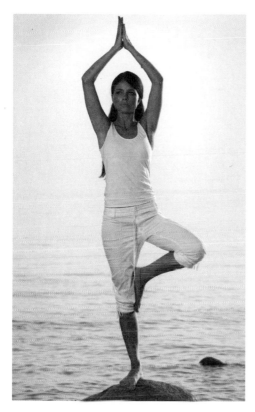

Above: Begin each practice with an open mind and be clear that this is time for you alone.

Your body is constantly responding to other circumstances. Just where your edge is varies from breath to breath, practice to practice, day to day. Rediscover your limit in every pose. Never take it for granted that you can stretch as far as you did yesterday. Never assume that you can't because you couldn't before.

It's irrelevant where your edge is in an asana. It is unimportant how far you stretch before you find it. Whether you reach your fingertips to your knees as you fold forward or whether you easily grasp your feet, let go of preconceptions of "good" or "proper" yoga. Seek instead just to find the point where you can learn about yourself.

Your psychological edge might be different to your physical edge. Respect both. Yoga should help you deal with life, not hinder

the process. Yoga asanas are a controlled means of exposing yourself to a difficult situation. They are meant to challenge you. They offer practice at mastering your reaction under stressful conditions. If you experience mental unease, absorb yourself in the breath. Should you find you are in a place that feels wrong, change it. If either your body or mind is telling you "no," don't push past it. Instead, as you do whenever circumstances change in your life, adjust. Be mentally flexible, too. Sensitively encourage yourself using your breath, but never force it.

YOUR INTENTION

Consider what you want to achieve with yoga. You might want to increase strength or flexibility, heal an ailment, find better body awareness, cope with stress, find inner peace, develop compassion, or explore your spirituality. Write down what it is you want, so that you will be clear and can form your practice around your goal. Also write how much time you can realistically expect to practice.

Yoga is not religious. Though yoga has been embraced by Hinduism, because they are both from Indian soil, there is nothing in the yoga texts that speaks of Hinduism. The writings do, however, recognize a divine principle, a universal energy. If you have a religious tradition that you find helpful, keep your personal god in mind. If not, consider your higher goals, or ideals that inspire you. Keeping in mind an energy greater than ourselves fosters our ability to attune to our higher selves.

At the start of your practice you might like to light a candle or an incense stick, offer a chant or prayer, or repeat an affirmation. You might look at a picture of your personal god, or a photo of someone inspirational with qualities you admire. Take time at the beginning to sit or lie quietly and access the stillness within. Be clear of your intent, but begin each practice with an open mind. Yoga, stilling the fluctuations of the mind, is an end point, but your practice is part of your journey, and a reward in itself.

Be clear that this is time for you alone. Close the door and turn off the phone. Let others know not to distract you. When a posture feels cumbersome and heavy, it will be less enjoyable. Bring mental lightness to your practice, too—enthusiasm always lightens the load. Practice with renewed effort when you feel lazy. If you feel you are a Type A overachiever, learn to ease off when your body requires it. Work honestly, with integrity, curiosity, and enthusiasm. Be joyful in your practice.

PHILOSOPHY

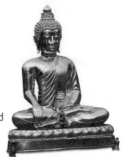

Hatha yoga consists of eight limbs of practices. They are not steps to be worked on one by one, but branches that can be explored, many at a time.

1 THE YAMAS

The yamas guide us in how we relate to others, our actions, thoughts, and speech. There are five listed in the Yoga-Sutra:

Ahimsa: Consideration for All Living Things

Often translated as nonviolence, ahimsa encompasses compassion for all beings. As well as obvious things like not killing insects or being abusive, this includes subtle things, such as avoiding gossip and mastering negative thoughts. Protect the environment by respecting nature and recycling. Develop kindness, patience, and tolerance for others and for yourself. Incorporate ahimsa in the way you eat and choose nourishing foods.

Satya: Right Communication

Satya deals with truthfulness and honesty in behavior and thought. It means refraining from deceptions or making a promise you cannot keep. If you are tempted to tell a "white" lie, be honest about your motivation. Is it to protect another or because of your inability to face an awkward situation? Lack of truth in any relationship doesn't build a stable foundation. Our task is to approach life with integrity and sincerity.

Asteya: Non-Covetousness

Despite its translation as non-stealing, asteya encompasses resisting the desire for things that don't belong to us, to avoid living in a state of unfulfilled wanting. Enjoy the simpler gifts of life. Asteya includes not taking that which is not freely given, such as not stealing another person's time by being late, or bullying someone into providing you with something you want. It means not taking the partner of another in an extramarital affair. Asteya encompasses giving credit where it is due.

Brahmacharya: Moderation in Our Actions

This has many interpretations, one of which is celibacy. Many spiritual traditions preach celibacy not because they consider sex bad, but so that energies can be used to uplift the Self. Celibacy

as a tool for discovering oneself can be a joyous, self-nurturing experience. An interpretation of brahmacharya might be being moderate in thoughts and actions. Channeling your sexuality with thought helps you to respect its power and use it with love.

Aparigraha: Non-Greediness

Consider your true needs—the less you need, the greater chance you have of being happy. Practice simplicity by paring down possessions to the essentials. Downsize the spiral of want and enjoy what you already have. Consider how easily you give to others. Appreciate that which is around you—good food, your health, uplifting conversation, a good friend.

2 THE NIYAMAS

The second limb, "niyamas," deals with our attitudes toward ourselves. The Yoga-Sutra lists five:

Saucha: Purity

Saucha is cleanliness of your physical body and surroundings. As mind and body influence each other, a healthy diet contributes to purity of mind. Purity in your home means not cluttering it with possessions. Cleanliness of living encompasses what you say, read, and watch on TV, and whom you associate with. Yoga cleanses the body with postures and breathing techniques. Clearing the mind through observance of the yamas and niyamas, and cleansing the spirit with meditation, allows for clarity of thinking.

Santosha: Contentment

Cultivate being satisfied with what you have, such as the knowledge that your basic needs are met, wonderful memories, your friendships, and your health. Appreciating these things helps to bring the happiness we seek. Santosha cultivates an uncomplaining approach toward what you don't have, rather than accepting what you have because you are too lazy to change. Embrace inner growth.

Tapas: Burning Enthusiasm

Tap means "to burn" or "to cook." Under this precept, you cook the raw ingredients of which you are composed to produce a beautiful dish. Tapas involves the self-control to live with good habits in all things, including work, food, drink, spirituality, thoughts, and wishes. Bring enthusiasm to all parts of your life and stay focused on your spiritual path.

Swadhyaya: Self-Study

Self-discovery demands a turning of the attention inward. Observe your responses under all circumstances. Whether you are relaxed or stressed, happy or sad, practice mindful self-reflection. Many people find keeping a journal helpful as a way of evaluating progress. Some choose therapy on their path to self-discovery; others attend spiritual classes. Read uplifting literature and other yoga books. As well as drawing your attention inward, extend your mind with philosophy and other studies that help you understand the world.

Ishvarapranidhana: Celebration of the Spiritual

Here we accept the existence of a higher intelligence. By honoring our relation to this all-knowing principle we surrender our small ego before a higher will, helping to fulfill our destiny. Remember that this omnipresent force always lies within. If you don't have a personal god, you may wish to celebrate an ideal.

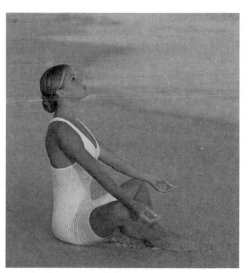

3 ASANA Postures

Asana, the third limb of yoga, is using physical postures as a method of self-study and exploration. Asana prepares the body and mind for meditation.

4 PRANAYAMA Control of the Prana

While breath comes automatically and unconsciously, pranayama is the conscious, deliberate regulation of the breath and prana, the vital force.

5 PRATYAHARA Withdrawal of the Senses

An example of this is when your hearing switches off from a dripping tap because you are engrossed in a book. While the senses are outward-looking, self-discovery involves turning the attention inward, subduing the senses. Listen to less radio and watch less TV; practice deep relaxation and meditation.

6 DHARANA Concentration

To maintain a mind undisturbed in its focus requires a certain mastery. Start small. Divide your dharana practice into small blocks of time—perhaps 30 seconds in an asana when you direct your mind to your body. During pranayama, direct it exclusively to the breath. By practicing you will become more accomplished.

7 DHYANA Meditation

Dhyana is a one-pointed mental focus around a single subject.

8 SAMADHI Bliss State

The highest level of experience and the goal of yoga—a bliss state where there is a sense of oneness. You reconnect with your essential purity, yet personal identity is not lost. The mind is mastered and thoughts are stilled in this trancelike state.

Left: *Through yoga, the body attains attractiveness to others, beauty, firmness, and unusual physical strength.*

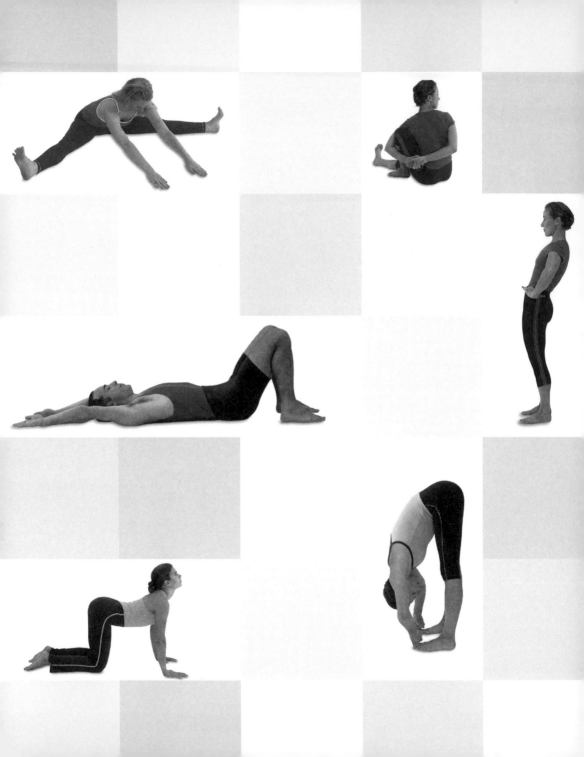

THE PRACTICE

STARTING THE JOURNEY

The following guidelines will help you get more out of your practice. Creating a special yoga practice area will reaffirm your commitment. You don't need much space, but make sure the area is warm, clean, and uncluttered.

Choose nonrestrictive clothes that you feel good in. Dress in layers to remain comfortable throughout your practice. Bare feet are best—wear socks only when your feet are cold. Intense practice in direct sunlight tends to be fatiguing, but relaxing in its warmth at the end is lovely. Practicing outside lets you commune with nature, but it can be more distracting than staying inside. It's a great idea to invest in a yoga mat. Apart from providing cushioning and a nonslip surface, it will make your mental commitment to your practice stronger. You will feel you can create a yoga space anywhere, simply by unrolling your mat.

Yoga works with prana, the vital force. Asana and pranayama practice bring this energy to the cells so they receive nourishment and can perform their functions and heal. When you eat, your energies are made available to the digestive system in preference to the other systems. So after a meal, leave a space before you practice. Wait one hour after having a piece of fruit or a juice. Wait three or four hours after a large meal. Hydrate yourself beforehand so you don't disturb yourself during the practice.

Be realistic when you decide how much time you would like to, and are able to, dedicate to your practice. It is helpful to make a mental commitment. Do your best to adhere to it, but don't think unkindly about yourself if you take a break. There has never been a yoga mat that has laid a guilt trip on someone who didn't use it for a while! Just work from where you are today. When you are short of time, practicing fewer poses

with complete attention is preferable to rushing through many poses. From time to time, look through this chapter to check on the exercises you may have been avoiding. Try to embrace them into your practice.

You don't need three-hour-long sessions of complicated asanas to practice "real" yoga. Sometimes one instant or a single breath is all you need to reconnect with yourself. Yoga practice is more than what you do on the mat. It is about how you live your life once you step off it, and that's 24 hours a day.

There are thousands of variations on hundreds of yoga poses, but don't let this intimidate you. Even if you feel like a human ironing board, you can benefit enormously from about 20 poses practiced regularly. It's like tending a garden. Left uncared for, the soil starts to dry up and the plants start to wither. Once the garden has reached a certain state, it's too late to rush in with the big hoses. Large amounts of water might be more than it can readily accept; instead it needs the kindness of water given little and often. If you have neglected your internal garden for a while, you'll need to practice in small, regular doses for it to grow and thrive.

Rather than focus on "perfecting" a posture as your measure of success in yoga, enjoy discovering your body and mind. Yoga is like life. It's a journey. Every yoga practice you have will be different, as you respond to internal and external conditions. Your thoughts change in a fraction of a second. The breath alters from second to second. How far you can stretch or hold a pose changes from minute to minute.

Empty your mind so that you can fully absorb the lessons of your practice. You never can predict just what they will be. If you are more adept, don't assume because you have practiced a posture a hundred times that you know everything about it. Keep the mind receptive and open to learning. Don't be impatient in your practice. Practice peacefully. Keep your mind sensitive. Overstraining the body will lessen your mental sensitivity. Some days you just might not feel like getting on your mat or doing breath work. Instead, your yoga practice might include reading something spiritually uplifting.

Take things easy during menstruation. It's a special time when it is nice to allow your energies to go inside. Avoid strong backbends and strong twists. Inverted postures mean the flow has to work against gravity, so avoid them. Women have a natural body clock that reminds them to practice slow, restful yoga regularly, but in my classes, men are allowed to "menstruate," too!

While yoga has helped the pregnancies and labors of countless women, it is not safe to begin during the first three months of pregnancy. Many poses need to be modified, so it's best to attend specialized classes during the second and third trimesters.

If you are suffering from a health condition or have an injury, seek guidance from an experienced yoga teacher or yoga therapist. Don't practice asanas or pranayama if you have a fever.

Attend some yoga classes. Yoga is so personal that each teacher will have something different to offer you. Teachers can give valuable feedback on your alignment and ideas for practice. Try teachers from several different traditions of yoga to find what suits you. Most yoga schools offer beginners' courses.

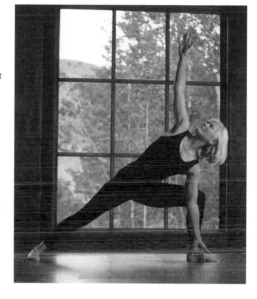

Above: *Practicing outside lets you commune with nature but may be more distracting than staying inside.*

Right and opposite: *Don't be impatient. Practice peacefully and keep your mind sensitive.*

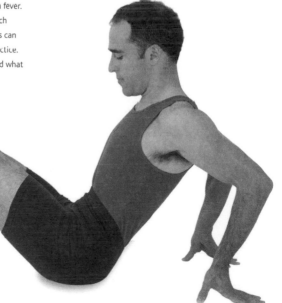

YOGA RELAXATION

Center yourself with a short relaxation before starting your asana practice, and always use it at the end of your practice. The final relaxation allows your body to integrate and consolidate the effects of the poses.

Imagine driving your car along the highway at high speed, for weeks on end. What would happen if you stopped only briefly to check the oil and water and refill the fuel? How long would your car last if subjected to days, weeks, and years of this? Now consider how you are driving your body. Like your car, your body will run better if given high-quality fuel and regular tune-ups. It will perform better for you when allowed to cool down with regular rest breaks.

Yoga asanas stir up the subtle energies (prana) of the body and the relaxation is the time that allows the prana to be directed to healing and reenergizing the system. You might feel as if nothing is happening and be tempted to skip this stage, but the final relaxation is hugely important and you risk losing valuable prana by missing it. Yoga relaxation allows you to emerge refreshed and brings your body, mind, and spirit back into balance. It is great after a long day, or while recovering from illness. Taking 20 minutes of conscious rest is enormously effective whenever you feel tired but need to keep working.

Many students gleefully exclaim "Sleep!" when relaxation time, yoga nidra, rolls around. Indeed, yoga nidra can be translated as yogic sleep, but remember that it is a conscious rest, requiring discipline. You practice being awake, yet free of body tension. After a strong session where you have really explored your boundaries, this active undoing comes more easily. As you take a break from external movement, cease fidgeting, and lie perfectly still, the mind becomes acutely sensitive. While you progressively let go of tension in the muscles, bones, organs, even the brain, you remain aware of the internal sensations. Whenever your thoughts stray, bring them back to your body. As the senses quieten and attention is turned inward, there is a heightened awareness. Quietening the body and mind, drawing the senses inward, and accessing your inner peace are steps along the path to meditation.

Lying still with your eyes closed looks easy. But if you tend to move through life at a frenetic pace, never ceasing to stop and

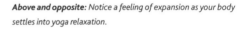

Above and opposite: *Notice a feeling of expansion as your body settles into yoga relaxation.*

take stock, falling into quietness can seem difficult. Conscious relaxation is an exercise in yielding. So many of us cling tenaciously to objects, people, habits, or attitudes. The principle of detachment is fundamental to Eastern philosophies. While you remain strongly attached to things, their loss will inevitably cause suffering. If you observe yourself holding onto things and accumulating material possessions, use yoga relaxation to consciously practice letting go. Physically and mentally permit yourself to release that grip and be just you, nothing else, lying on the floor. As you actively undo, you let your defenses down and accept the sense of vulnerability inherent in allowing surrender.

Try making a fist with one hand and keeping it clenched for ten seconds. Now relax the fist and compare the feelings in the two hands. Most likely you'll feel more sensations in the hand that was clenched. As you seek to find the edge in each posture, you will be fully occupying both muscles and mind. Once the tension is released, a lingering awareness remains. The same principle applies in yoga relaxation. When you have extended your body to its limit, you'll notice how your awareness of internal sensations deepens, because your mind has been completely engrossed in your practice. It will very easily let go into deep relaxation.

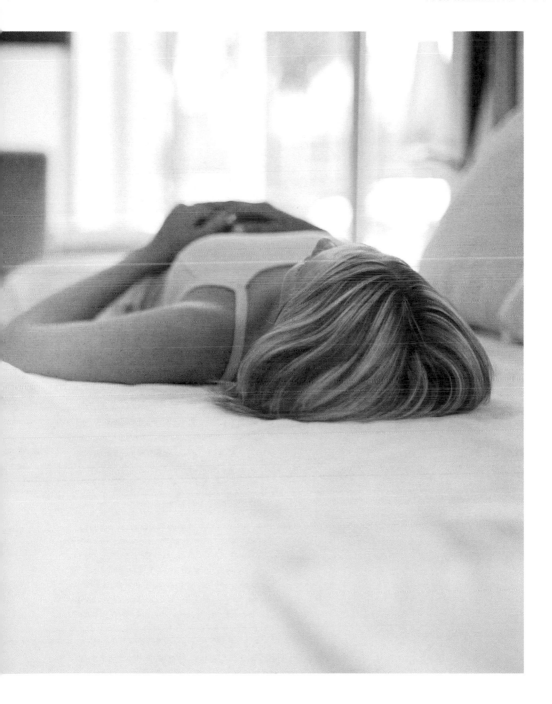

GETTING COMFORTABLE FOR RELAXATION

Help yourself let go by becoming perfectly physically comfortable. Any of these modifications to the basic supine position may be helpful. *See* page 26 for how to make a "breathing bed." The Child Pose is useful whenever you need to relax during your practice or throughout your day.

USING A PILLOW

Find the best position for your head by having a friend observe you as you lie on your back. Ideally, your chin and forehead will be at an equal height from the floor. If your chin is higher than your forehead, the back of the neck will tend to shorten. Many people don't need more than a thinly folded blanket to soften the floor for the head. However, if you find your chin juts up higher than your forehead when you are lying, make a pillow.

If the forehead is too high, the throat will feel constricted. Use a folded blanket to bring your chin and forehead level.

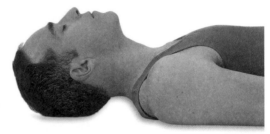

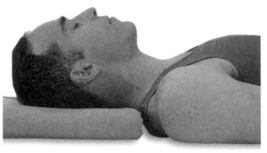

MAKING A NECK PILLOW

Fold a blanket three times and roll it up about halfway. Wedge this securely under your neck, right up to shoulder level. Experiment with the amount of roll. Your neck should feel very snug with the roll supporting its natural curve. Usually the chin juts out a little, so fold the remaining flap down to cushion and lift the back of the head.

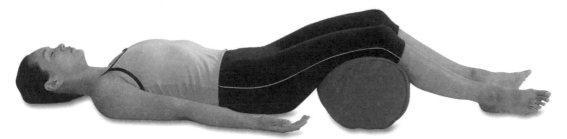

SUPPORTING THE LOWER BACK

This support lets the lower back soften down closer to the floor, and those with lower back problems find it useful. Place large rolled cushions or a bolster under your knees, and do a small pelvic tilt to flatten the lower back toward the floor. Your lower back will still curve up away from the floor, but as you then lie and let go, you will feel it ease out and release a little. If you don't have any props, then bend your knees, place your feet just wider than body width, and lean the knees in together.

COVER UP

When you relax deeply, your body temperature drops dramatically. It is impossible to let go completely when you are cold. Unless it is the height of summer, cover your whole body with a shawl or blanket.

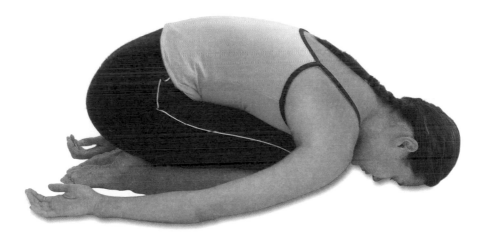

CHILD POSE

Sit on your heels with your knees together. Fold forward over your thighs. Rest your forehead to the floor and drape your arms around you. Close your eyes and let go of any tension. Enjoy the reassuring massage of the belly pressing down into the thighs with each inhalation. For high blood pressure, or if your buttocks stay high in the air and you feel as if you are nosediving, rest your forehead on a pad of folded blankets. Alternatively, stack your fists one on top of the other to rest your forehead on.

GUIDED RELAXATION IN SAVASANA CORPSE POSE

While this pose looks like the easiest of all the yoga asanas, it is actually one of the hardest to master. While the body lets go, the mind must stay alert, observing the relaxation process, before finally surrendering to rest. The final relaxation allows your body to settle and the effects of your hatha yoga practice to consolidate. Spend about five minutes working through the body to exaggerate the tension in your muscles, section by section. This raises the level of awareness so you can better surrender to complete relaxation. A nice way to practice Savasana is to make a tape of these instructions, with plenty of pauses, or have a friend read them aloud.

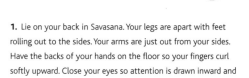

1. Lie on your back in Savasana. Your legs are apart with feet rolling out to the sides. Your arms are just out from your sides. Have the backs of your hands on the floor so your fingers curl softly upward. Close your eyes so attention is drawn inward and you become sensitized to your inner environment.

EXPLORE

As a general rule, for every 30 minutes of asana practice, practice at least five minutes of Savasana. For a 90-minute practice, allow 15 minutes of relaxation at the end.

But you don't need to practice any asanas to reward yourself with Savasana. Practice relaxation whenever you feel tired. Instead of taking a daytime nap, refresh with 20 minutes of Savasana.

2. Scrunch your toes and flex your feet. Next, spread out your toes and point the feet strongly. Then relax your feet.

3. Lift your right leg 2 in (5 cm) in the air. Briefly tense all the muscles in that leg and then release them, letting the leg fall to the floor. Do the same with the left leg.

4. Clench your buttocks for a few seconds so your hips rise slightly. Release. Feel the heaviness of your lower body.

5. Tighten the muscles along the length of the spine and press the tips of your shoulders into the floor. Puff your chest up and tighten your abdominal muscles. Then exhale and relax the muscles, let the chest release downward, and allow the tension to flow out of the body.

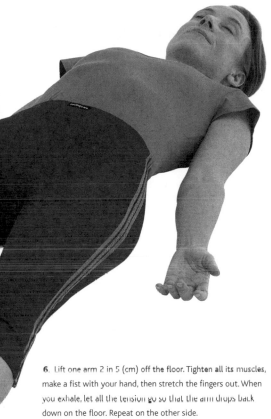

10. Press the chin to the throat so you feel the back of the neck lengthening, then release it by softening all the neck muscles. So that you can commit to lying perfectly still for the next ten minutes, mentally check your position and adjust anything you need to. Just like during meditation, any outer movement will distract you from your inner world.

11. Become aware of the whole body being heavy and relaxed. Your body wants to be comfortable. It is in its natural state. The bones feel heavy. All the muscles are relaxed. The internal organs are free of tension. Even the tongue is relaxed. As the body releases and feels heavier, the breath lightens and feels more delicate. The brain surrenders any worries and is content, enjoying this peaceful and tranquil moment. Give permission for your emotional body to let go, too. While the body relaxes, the mind stays present, observing. Finally, completely stop trying to "do." Let go of any psychological effort at all. Now rest.

6. Lift one arm 2 in 5 (cm) off the floor. Tighten all its muscles, make a fist with your hand, then stretch the fingers out. When you exhale, let all the tension go so that the arm drops back down on the floor. Repeat on the other side.

7. Lift the shoulders to the ears into a shrug and then release them back down and toward the hips.

8. Tighten all the facial muscles. Lose your inhibitions—no one is watching you! Clench your jaw muscles, squeeze the eyes tightly shut, and frown. Then widen everything out and apart. Open your eyes and roll the eyeballs back, open your mouth and stick the tongue as far out toward the chin as you can. Finally, exhale with a sigh and relax the face. Feel all the skin on the face soften and any wrinkles smooth out.

9. This time without tensing, gently drop your right ear to the floor. Take a few long breaths and become aware of the stretch on the left side of the neck. Inhale, bring the head to the center and drop the left ear to the floor for a few breaths before bringing the head to center again.

12. You will intuitively know when it's time to come out of the relaxation. Begin to move the fingers and toes as you focus back on the body. Take your arms overhead along the floor and stretch up through the body, enlivening everything from fingertips to toes. When you are ready, roll over onto your side and allow the eyes to open in their own time.

EXPLORE

Your tongue is a huge muscle, attaching deep into the throat. There's much more of it than you can see when you stick it out. It usually sits touching the roof of the mouth. Instead, release it down so it floats in the center of the mouth. This relaxes the whole mouth, throat area, and face. Observe whether this allows other more distant parts of the body to release, too.

REVITALIZING RELAXATION

To make a "breathing bed," fold one to three blankets so that they are 8 in (20 cm) wide and longer than your torso. Lie over them with your buttocks on the floor and legs a little apart. The more blankets you use, the more the chest will feel it is opening, so experiment with what feels best for you. Use another blanket as a pillow so that the head is higher than the chest. Take your legs apart and let your arms rest out to the sides.

Lie on your back and lift your head for a moment to look down your body to make sure you are perfectly symmetrical. After checking that you feel completely comfortable, begin to breathe deeply and rhythmically. As you inhale, visualize prana being drawn in through the nostrils down to your solar plexus. As you exhale it swirls around your center. With each inhalation, draw this pranic energy down to the solar plexus so that it spirals around, filling up the whole torso. Each long, deep inhalation draws in more prana. While you are giving yourself the gift of vibrant energy, remember to keep the exhalations slow and steady. The full exhalation empties the lungs, allowing you to inhale this revitalizing force deeply and consciously.

From the center of the torso the spiral enlarges to cover the whole body. The outer part of the spiral reaches to circle over the head, fingertips, and toes. Let yourself become the breath. With this positive energy you become enthusiastic about life and your tasks. You gain the energy to fulfill them. Stay here as long as you need to.

When it is time to awaken, start moving your body and stretch a little. Feel so revitalized that the eyes blink open by themselves, as if powered by the energy within.

WHITE LIGHT

To stay true to your inner self and protect yourself from being harmed or feeling drained by others, visualize yourself surrounded with glowing white light.

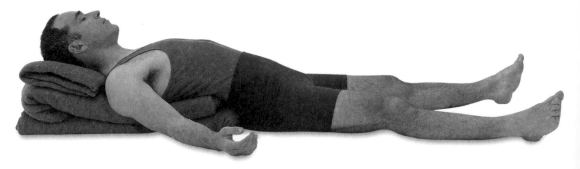

HEALING VISUALIZATION

The use of color is a therapeutic branch on its own. White light gives strength of spirit, clarity, and protection. Black, the absence of light, brings qualities of strength, power, evolution, and transition. Yellow, the color of the intellect, is uplifting and joyful. Red fosters courage, warmth, and assertiveness. Orange is used for creativity, optimism, and tolerance. Sky blue is linked to sincerity, peace, honesty, and organizational abilities. Indigo promotes mental calmness and lessens attachment to material possessions. Violet fosters self-esteem and confidence, and dissolves the ego. Emerald green brings physical and emotional harmony and is recharging. Each chakra (see page 152) has a related color.

Choose a color to which you feel intuitively drawn. As you lie quietly in Savasana, draw this color into any area of your body you would like to heal. With each inhalation, the color becomes clearer and brighter. It forms a dense core and, from there, begins to expand outward. In your mind's eye, visualize it expanding to fill the whole body: see it clearly filling your heart, a center for healing and unconditional love that keeps enlarging it. Take several minutes, allowing it to spill over to fill the whole body all the way down the legs to the toes, and all the way down the arms to the fingertips. Breathe this color up into your head. It fills your brain, the backs of your eyes, all the crevices behind the face. You happily accept the healing energy that your special color offers. You may like to send goodwill or healing to loved ones. Before you complete this exercise, mentally seal your color and its particular qualities in your body.

CREATING A SANCTUARY

Think of a place where you know you can feel completely at ease. It could be a real place you have visited or seen or else an imaginary paradise—a special sanctuary where you feel completely safe, protected, and nurtured. It might be next to a still, deep pond, near the ocean, in a lush green forest, or by a flickering fireplace in a wonderful home. Now, as you lie in Savasana, visualize yourself from above. From lying on the floor, visualize your body coming up to standing, and start on a pleasant trip toward your special place. Feel the sun on your skin and the breeze in your hair. Listen to the calls of the birds

and the other sounds around, like leaves in the gentle wind or a babbling brook. In time, you arrive at your special place and settle yourself down to sit in a meditative position. Visualize yourself sitting with eyes closed and a peaceful mind. Your sanctuary gives nourishment, and you are safe to relax completely. Continue to see yourself sitting quietly. Know that your sanctuary is always there when you need it. You just need to take the time to access it.

When it is time to come back, rouse yourself from sitting and take the journey back to where you are lying, until you can see yourself on the floor again. Begin to tune in to the sounds around you. Feel the touch of the clothes on your skin, then roll over and sit up slowly.

EXPLORE

Often mental anxiety around a health problem builds up. This creates more tension and pain. Practice directing calm, focused, accepting thoughts to that area. If only for a short time, separate yourself from your usual response to this challenge. Empty yourself of anxiety. Mentally send your breath to the area to release, soothe, and heal.

BUILDING AWARENESS

The following exercises are good ways to reconnect with yourself at the start of a practice session.

ABSORB YOURSELF IN YOUR BREATH

The stresses of day-to-day life can create different layers of breathing over our free, natural breath. This exercise will help you reconnect with your natural breath. Keep it simple. You are not aiming to go anywhere. You don't have to "do" anything. This is not a new technique, but rather a process of undoing. There is no need for effort, pushing, or wanting. There is no search to attain the "perfect" breath. Instead, let it unravel. Often we are guided by our mental intelligence, but instead, let your instinctual natural physical intelligence take over as you unravel. Your body is what is breathing, not your mind. Your mind, relinquishing control, learns to move out of the way and becomes merely the accepting observer. Come back to this exercise regularly. Make sure that you allow at least 20 minutes for it.

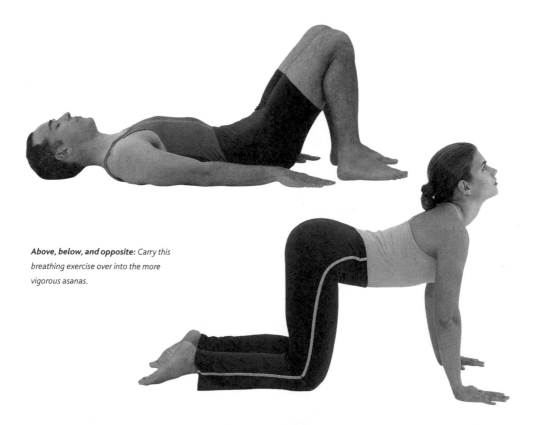

Above, below, and opposite: Carry this breathing exercise over into the more vigorous asanas.

Lie on your back with your knees bent and feet flat on the floor. Swivel your feet so your big toes are closer together than your inner heels, then lean your knees in together, so holding them in place is effortless. Have your arms out by your sides, palms facing down. Close your eyes. Give your full attention to your breathing. Can you feel where the breath originates? Observe which part of your body moves first as you breathe in. What happens next? Observe the sequence of your body's movement when you inhale. Feel what happens to the lower and upper abdomen. How do the ribcage and chest work? Can you feel anything happening at the back? What happens to the shoulders, throat, face, and nostrils? Does anything change at the pelvis?

Absorb yourself completely in your breath. You are your breath and your breath is you. It rises and falls with the rhythm of ocean waves. How do you accept your inhalation? How do you feel the expansion? Now turn your attention to the out breath. From where do you exhale? Which part of the body begins the movement? Where does your exhalation end? Are the movements in the torso as clearly demarcated as in your inhalation? Can you feel a consolidation of energy? Accept the support of the earth each time. Don't shrink, but let yourself sink.

Count the length of your in and out breaths. Which is longer? Does one come more easily to you? Become aware of the quality of your breath. Is it shallow or deep? How rhythmic does it feel? Does it feel smooth or coarse? Is it graceful and round, or are there some parts that feel jerky or jagged? Does it feel soothing?

Often we don't breathe out fully, but hurry on to the next inhalation. Take the time to follow the entire length of your exhalation. Stay with it. Patiently wait until it is finished before you take your next breath. It takes some time to release all the used air from the alveoli. There is no need to tighten any muscles to "squeeze" the last air out. Just be patient and let it keep on flowing. Whenever you feel you are trying too hard, release the effort.

Now become aware of the time at the end of the exhalation, before the next inhalation begins. There is a brief moment before your lungs call for air. Don't grab for the next breath. Sink into this natural pause and enjoy it. It is a moment of tranquillity, as still as a deep, calm pond. The exhalation disappears into it, and then the stillness gives birth to the inhalation. As you observe this stillness, you may find the pause lengthening naturally.

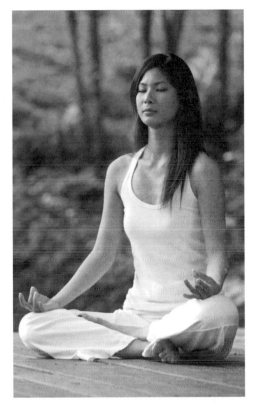

Now attune yourself to what happens at the top of the inhalation, before you feel the need to exhale. There is another pause, another precious moment. It is a full silence that you can relax into. As you let yourself sink into this moment, it will expand.

These pauses give rise to a breath in four parts: a releasing exhalation; a still pause; the gift of a new inhalation; and a pause. Become absorbed in a meditative way in each part of your breath. No two breaths are the same. Make friends with your breath and get to know each part intimately.

Before you roll over to sit up, take some time to observe the effects this exercise has had on your mind. You have learned a new skill to quieten the mind. You have developed your self-awareness, and practiced being absorbed in the present moment.

Have a friend read the instructions with plenty of pauses to allow you to explore.

1 CHEST-OPENING EXERCISE

AWARENESS OF THE BREATH

Channeling the breath into movement is centering
and helps maintain a steady rhythmic breath.

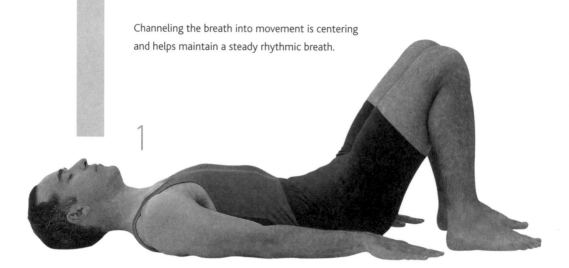

1. Lie on your back with your knees bent and your hands
palms down on the floor. To begin, exhale fully.

2. While you inhale, raise your arms (2a)
overhead until the backs of your hands come to
rest on or near the floor (2b). Energize your arms
so that they extend and lift out of your
shoulders to flow through a large arc.

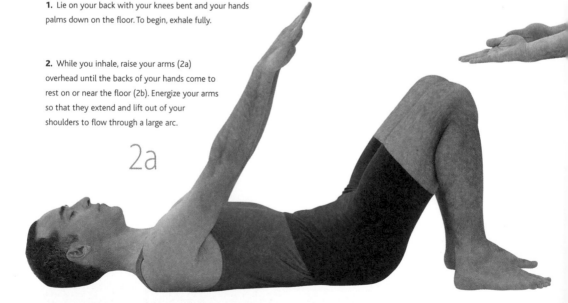

3. Exhale and raise your arms to bring them back to the starting position. With eyes closed, continue moving between these two movements. Time the movement to follow your breath, not the other way around. Because you keep the flow of air in and out through the nostrils at a steady rate, your arm movements are also constant and graceful.

2b

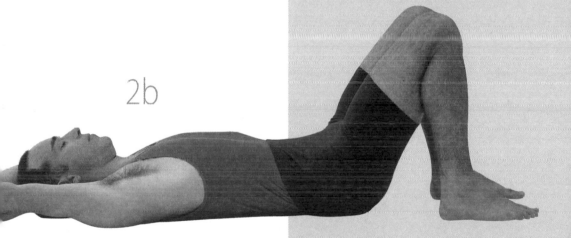

4. Now become aware of how your torso moves in relation to the arm movements. As you inhale and raise the arms, feel the natural life of the upper back as it lifts away from the floor. Rest with your arms overhead for several breaths. The upper back will ground more into the floor, and your chest will naturally open and promote a lovely full inhalation. Each time you exhale and bring your arms down, tune into the softening down that happens in the torso as it releases into the earth. Moving slowly, with awareness, bring your attention to your pelvis. Can you feel the gentle tilting backward and forward with each part of the breath? Take some more time, unhurriedly observing the movements of the body in response to the breath.

BIRALASANA Cat Pose

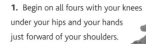

This exercise brings awareness and flexibility to the entire length of the spine. The key to awareness is to move slowly. Practice patience and keep an enquiring mind.

1. Begin on all fours with your knees under your hips and your hands just forward of your shoulders.

2. Inhale and concave your back. Move your breastbone forward and up, and raise your tailbone up. Keep the back of your neck long as you gaze upward. Press the palms evenly against the floor and avoid slumping into the shoulders.

3. As you exhale, round your back. Your upper back arches naturally in this way, so place particular awareness on the movement of the lower back as it follows this new curve upward as you tuck your pelvis under. Observe how your shoulder blades spread apart and the skin between them stretches. As you finish your exhalation, move your chin toward your breastbone.

4. Repeat ten more rounds, arching and rounding in time to your breath. Accentuate the curve so it is deeper each time.

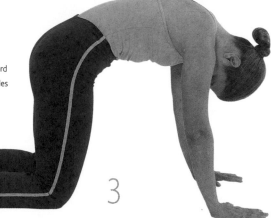

2

3

SUKHASANA FORWARD FOLD

CROSS-LEGGED FORWARD FOLD

Sukha means "content" or "happy." Spending a few minutes letting
yourself soften into this pose is a centering way to start your practice.

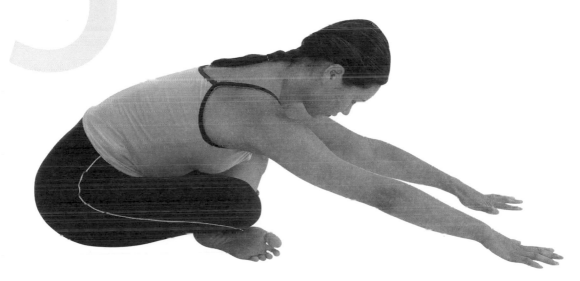

1. Sit in a simple cross-legged position. To work deeper into the
hips, slide your heels away from each other so that they rest
under the knees. Then take the feet forward so the shins are in a
horizontal line.

2. Become aware of the sitting bones in contact with the floor.
This base will act as your anchor as you stretch forward. Place
your fingertips on the floor just in front of your legs. Now
lengthen the sides of the torso from hips to armpits. Use several
breaths to let this releasing take place. When you feel ready,
creep the hands away. Work with your breath as you take one or
two minutes to slide the hands forward in stages. Only drop your
forehead down to the floor if your front ribs come to lie on your
legs. Then repeat with the legs crossed the other way.

EXPLORE

Don't become mentally lazy. Stay aware. If you are performing
the pose automatically, you might just stay at the point you
initially reached. When you use longer holds in a pose, often
you will find you can go much deeper and extend yourself to
your new edge.

4 ROLL DOWNS

Working through this sequence will allow you to learn about how undoing, rather than active doing, can deepen a pose.

1. Stand in Tadasana (*see* page 38) with your feet hip-width apart. You are going to take several breaths to fold forward by rolling down the spine.

2. As you exhale, drop your head forward (2a). Feel how the shoulders want to follow. Release your knees so that they bend slightly. On your next exhalation let the shoulders go and the upper back round more. Your arms hang down vertically, dangling passively out of their sockets (2b). Continue exhaling and rolling down the back in stages, leading with the head. Your knees will bend more the farther you roll down. Take as many breaths as you need to release all the way down.

EXPLORE

Repeat the same process, rolling down to each side in turn. Indulge by giving yourself plenty of time.

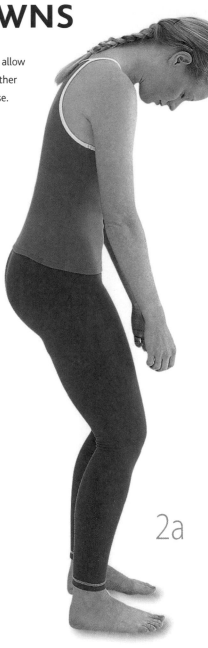

2a

3. Even though your legs are working, your upper body is dangling, hanging out of the hips. Bring a rag-doll quality to the upper body. Move your awareness to the shoulders and relax them fully so the arms hang loose. Relax the back of the neck so the crown of the head is the closest part of the head to the floor.

4. Take several rounds of breathing, observing the movements intrinsically related to the breath. As you inhale there is a lifting energy in the core of the body. If your knees are bent enough, a small lengthening occurs from pubic bone to throat. As you exhale, your ribs will fall closer to your thighs.

5. When it's time to come up, keep the knees bent and, over several breaths, roll up slowly through the spine, as if you are stacking each vertebra on top of the last. Exhale; release the arms down to the sides.

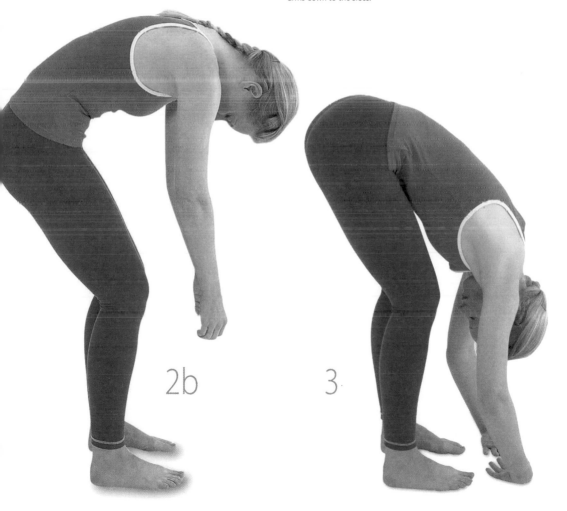

2b

3

STANDING POSTURES

Within the standing postures you find side bends, backbends, forward bends, twists, and balances. With the exception of the inverted positions, they embody the effects of all the other groups of yoga postures.

Regular practice of the standing poses is a great start for all yogis. They increase strength and flexibility in equal parts. As they extend and integrate the whole body, they help correct imbalances of the vertebral column. They develop grace, endurance, perseverance, and concentration. They help you to feel energetic and enthusiastic.

Because they involve the whole body, they warm you in preparation for the other poses. Since they are expansive poses, you can more easily see the directions of energy extension as the arms and legs extend from the spine. You can use these energies to give your poses a lightness. Over time, these poses will even help to bring the spring back into flatfeet.

In order to achieve anything in life, we need somewhere to extend from. Standing postures let us develop roots. They allow us to examine how we "stand on our own two feet" and how to "stand our ground." They help us establish a firm base to ensure the upper body is well supported. In standing poses we play off stability with extension as we practice radiating from this steady base.

EXPLORE

Stay in your habitual standing position for long enough without moving until the sensations begin to intensify. Then take this feedback and see what you need to do to realign and prevent the discomfort coming to those points. Do this when you are sitting in your habitual way in your favorite armchair, too.

CAUTION

Avoid standing poses in acute cases of asthma, colitis, nervous disorders, or cardiac problems. Don't jump in or out of the poses if you are pregnant, menstruating, or if you have back or knee injuries.

EXPLORE

Sit on the floor and give your feet a little massage first. Do small karate chops on the soles of the feet. Make loose fists and do some light pounding. Rub your hands briskly over the feet using the friction to build warmth. Now you might find it easier to become aware of how your feet contact the earth.

FROM THE GROUND UP

1. Have a look at your feet. How are the arches? Do they lift up or do they collapse downward to produce flatfeet or knock-knees? How are your toes? Are they squashed together from wearing tight shoes? Are they white with tension as they cling to the ground? Ungrip the toes by lifting them and spreading them apart. Keeping them stretched away, place them down on the floor.

2. Stand erect and feel where the heaviness comes into the feet. Where is the weight centered? Is there more weight placed on the balls of the feet, or the heels? Is one foot taking more weight than another? Rock back and forth to find your center. Keeping the feet on the floor, transfer the weight from left to right and back several times to home in on the center of grounding. Lean in all directions in a large circle. Then slowly reduce the size of the circle until you find your centered point.

3. Mentally soften the soles of your feet. Spread the skin. Let your breath come into the feet. They widen and soften with each exhalation. Visualize roots growing downward. By earthing the feet, the rest of the body is free to expand and lengthen.

FROM THE PELVIS UP

1. Anterior tilt. Stand with hands on your hips, fingers pointing forward, so that your index fingers rest on top of the hip bones and press into the waist. Tilt your pelvis forward, just as if it were a basin and you were tipping water out of the front of it. Your fingers will point down and your thumbs will lift. Feel how the curve in your lower back accentuates and your chest lifts a bit. This action makes the knees push back, too.

2. Posterior tilt. Now tilt the pelvis the other way, as if you were pouring out water from the back. Your fingers will rise up and your thumbs move down. Your lower back curve will flatten and the fronts of your knees will move forward. The chest tends to slump, abdominal length shortens and shoulders roll forward. Feel how this affects your neck, too. If you are not sure, exaggerating the movements might help.

3. Come back to the center, so your pelvis is not tipped forward or back, but centered. Take time to feel how it is mentally, comparing it to your normal way of standing.

By taking time to move in between the anterior and posterior pelvic tilt positions, you will become familiar with the trickle-on effects of them on the rest of your body. A truly centered pelvis would actually be too unstable to carry us well, so people tend to have a pelvis tilted either one way or the other. Ideally, this position would be just off center, rather than strongly so. Still standing, find a more centered position for your pelvis. Observe how your body feels when compared to your normal way of carrying yourself. Slowly move around the room like this, exploring new possibilities for carriage and movement.

ELONGATING THE CURVES OF THE SPINE

1. Stand with your back to a wall or doorframe. Take your feet about 1 ft (30 cm) away from the wall, and a little bit apart, with the outside edges of the feet parallel. Lean against the wall so your body contacts the wall at the sacrum and the thoracic curve. The small of the back (lumbar region) will arch away from the wall. How easily the back of your head comes to the wall depends on the curves of your spine. If your upper back is very flat, your throat will feel constricted. If your upper back is very rounded, it will be more difficult to bring your head comfortably to the wall. If your chin juts out and the back of the neck shortens, find a midway position for the head. Gently bring your floating ribs down, so they don't jut out. Don't bend your knees. Bring the tops of the thighs back slightly so the front of the groin opens.

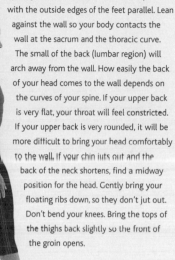

2. The spine is most effectively lengthened by undoing, rather than doing. Take plenty of time to release so the spine can elongate upward. If you actively work the muscles that run along the spine, then they will contract and actually shorten the vertebral column. Likewise, there is no need to raise the shoulders to grow taller. Instead, let go with each exhalation. Let your tailbone be heavy so that it eases down toward the floor. Keep your weight well grounded through your feet. As you continue to lengthen, feel the very small movements that ripple along the spine in connection with the breath. Are there any areas of your spine that feel blocked? Concentrate on softening the tight spots. When you move away from the wall, walk softly around the room, feeling the effects of this exercise.

TADASANA MOUNTAIN POSE

This pose connects you to both earth and sky. It is a wonderful exercise in centering and being able to respond to situations from a solid base. Begin and end each of the standing poses with this centered position. Use it as a chance to hear your body's feedback to what happened in the last pose. Although you appear steady as a mountain, you are not as hard as a rock in this pose. Externally your mountain is still, but bring it alive from the inside, where it feels dynamic and alive, responding to every breath. Practice Tadasana whenever possible throughout the day.

1. Stand with your feet a little less than hip-width apart, with the outside edges of your feet parallel. Follow the instructions for softening the feet on page 36. While your feet ground downward, move your awareness to your legs and get a sense of extending up toward the sky, starting at the ankle joints. Let your pelvis be in a neutral position (*see* previous page). The spine, supported by the pelvis, is freed to lengthen upward. It is perfectly possible to stand erect and be relaxed at the same time. Exhale tension out of the spine so it is released to grow taller. Feel your arms dangling from the shoulder sockets. Let them hang, and completely let go. As your shoulders soften down, the neck and head float and rise out of them. Release the mouth, tongue, and jaw. Observe whether this allows other more distant parts of the body to release, too. Bring a sense of weightlessness to the head. Visualize it as a helium-filled balloon on the end of a stick, your spine. Mentally sweep over your body to see where the heaviness is.

2. Check in with your breathing. Release the diaphragm muscle. Take slow, deep, steady breaths. Feel the ripple-like effect of each breath on the spine. Quite different from an upward movement induced by muscle tension, feel the lifting energy with each inhalation. Your body has its own innate intelligence. Be curious! Follow your breath to feel where it lets your body open and expand. Explore any subtle effects that your exhalation has on it.

PRASARITA PADOTTANASANA

WIDE LEG STRETCH

In asanas the arms and legs often act as levers to work the spine. But make sure they work with the rest of your body and breath, not forcefully overriding them.

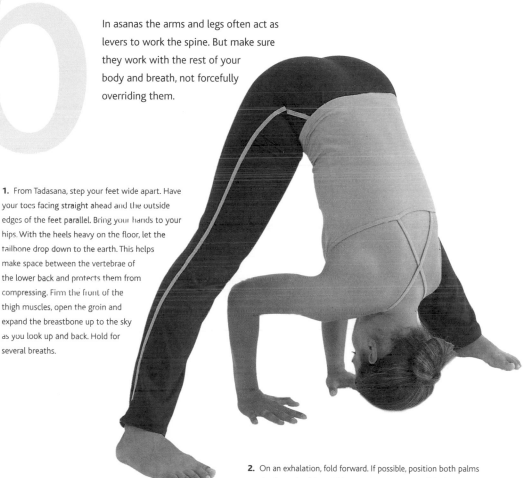

1. From Tadasana, step your feet wide apart. Have your toes facing straight ahead and the outside edges of the feet parallel. Bring your hands to your hips. With the heels heavy on the floor, let the tailbone drop down to the earth. This helps make space between the vertebrae of the lower back and protects them from compressing. Firm the front of the thigh muscles, open the groin and expand the breastbone up to the sky as you look up and back. Hold for several breaths.

EXPLORE

Interlace your fingers behind your back and take your arms overhead. Firm your front thigh muscles as your thumbs move toward the floor.

2. On an exhalation, fold forward. If possible, position both palms on the floor, shoulder-width apart, upper arms parallel. If you are still developing your hamstring flexibility, bend your knees if necessary to bring your fingertips to the floor. Unhunch shoulders by sliding the shoulder blades up toward the hips. Walk the hands back as they lever you deeper into a forward bend. When it is time to come up, bring your hands back onto your hips. Firm the thigh and abdominal muscles and inhale to come up.

VIRABHADRASANA I WARRIOR I

This all-involving pose works the arms and legs, strengthens the back, and opens the chest.

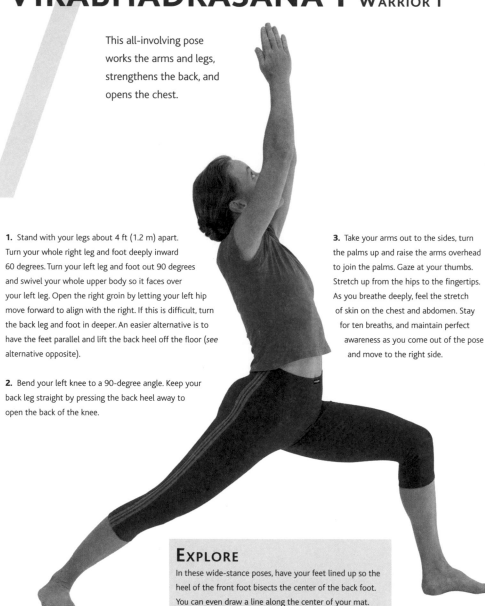

1. Stand with your legs about 4 ft (1.2 m) apart. Turn your whole right leg and foot deeply inward 60 degrees. Turn your left leg and foot out 90 degrees and swivel your whole upper body so it faces over your left leg. Open the right groin by letting your left hip move forward to align with the right. If this is difficult, turn the back leg and foot in deeper. An easier alternative is to have the feet parallel and lift the back heel off the floor (*see* alternative opposite).

2. Bend your left knee to a 90-degree angle. Keep your back leg straight by pressing the back heel away to open the back of the knee.

3. Take your arms out to the sides, turn the palms up and raise the arms overhead to join the palms. Gaze at your thumbs. Stretch up from the hips to the fingertips. As you breathe deeply, feel the stretch of skin on the chest and abdomen. Stay for ten breaths, and maintain perfect awareness as you come out of the pose and move to the right side.

EXPLORE

In these wide-stance poses, have your feet lined up so the heel of the front foot bisects the center of the back foot. You can even draw a line along the center of your mat.

ALTERNATIVE: HEEL LIFTED

An easier alternative for beginners is to have the feet
parallel and lift up the back heel off the floor. If you have
trouble balancing, step the front foot a little to the side.
Sometimes people unconsciously hunch their shoulders
when attempting to press their palms together. Until your
shoulder flexibility develops, take your palms apart and
arms parallel and check if this releases it. If you still feel
"bad" shoulder tension, then lower your arms ten or 20
degrees forward, with attention to spreading
the shoulder blades well apart.

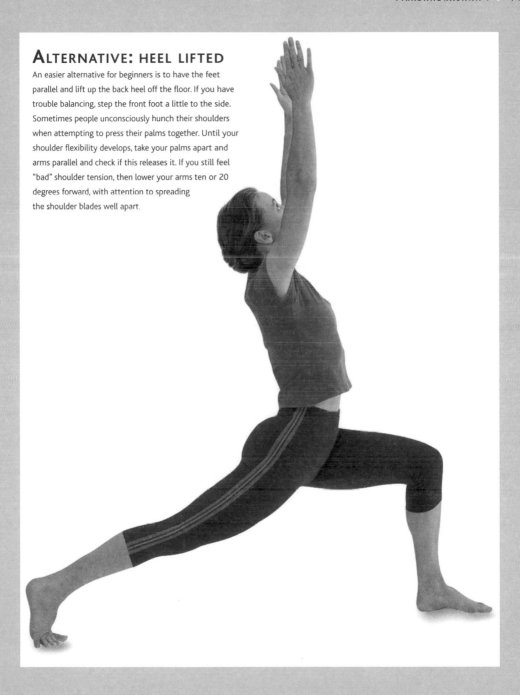

VIRABHADRASANA II WARRIOR II

8

As if you were aiming a bow and arrow at your target, maintain a perfect mental focus over your middle finger. Strong legs give self-reliance and independence and the raised head, fearlessness.

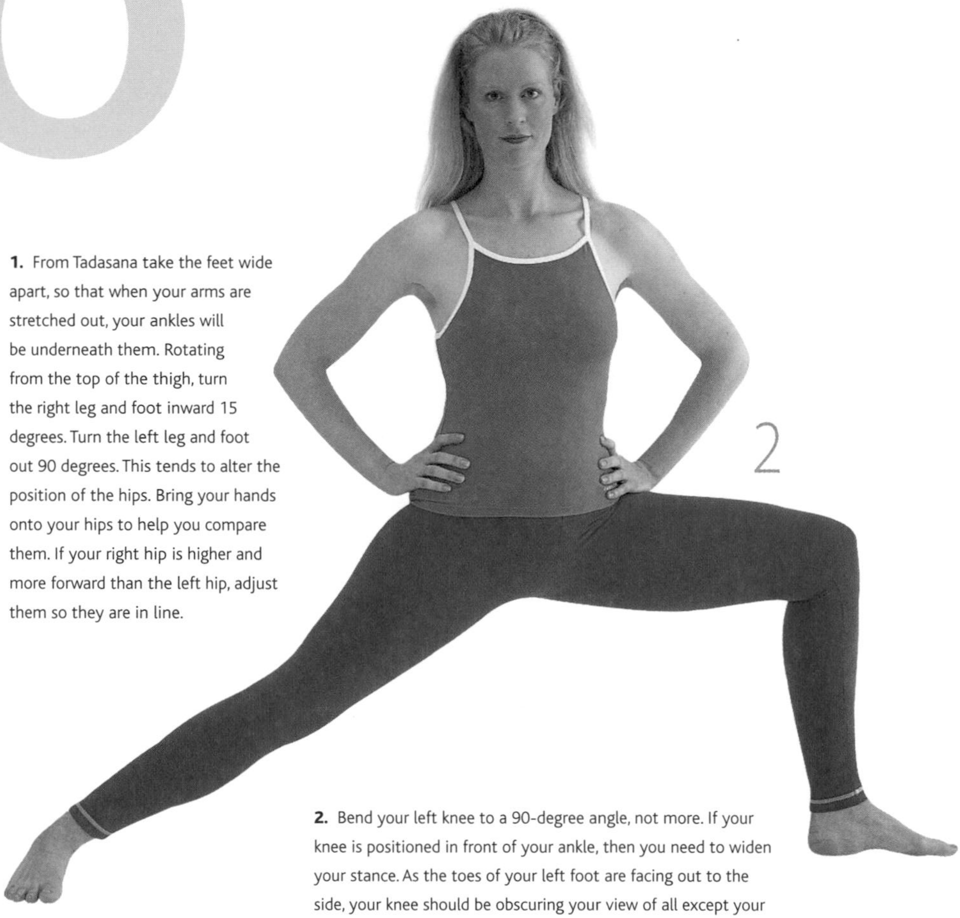

1. From Tadasana take the feet wide apart, so that when your arms are stretched out, your ankles will be underneath them. Rotating from the top of the thigh, turn the right leg and foot inward 15 degrees. Turn the left leg and foot out 90 degrees. This tends to alter the position of the hips. Bring your hands onto your hips to help you compare them. If your right hip is higher and more forward than the left hip, adjust them so they are in line.

2

2. Bend your left knee to a 90-degree angle, not more. If your knee is positioned in front of your ankle, then you need to widen your stance. As the toes of your left foot are facing out to the side, your knee should be obscuring your view of all except your big toe. Look down the front of your torso to check that the ribs on both sides are even.

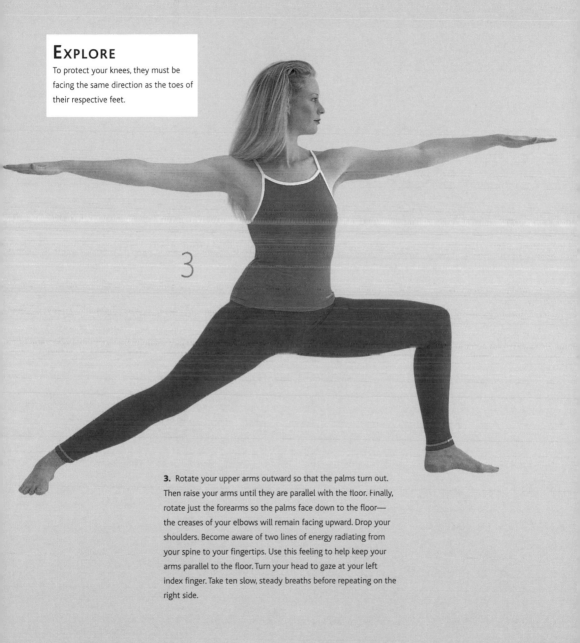

EXPLORE

To protect your knees, they must be facing the same direction as the toes of their respective feet.

3

3. Rotate your upper arms outward so that the palms turn out. Then raise your arms until they are parallel with the floor. Finally, rotate just the forearms so the palms face down to the floor—the creases of your elbows will remain facing upward. Drop your shoulders. Become aware of two lines of energy radiating from your spine to your fingertips. Use this feeling to help keep your arms parallel to the floor. Turn your head to gaze at your left index finger. Take ten slow, steady breaths before repeating on the right side.

TRIKONASANA

TRIANGLE POSE

9

This pose has five rays of energy: two arms stretching away, two legs stretching out and down, and a fifth line running from the tailbone as it extends toward the crown of the head.

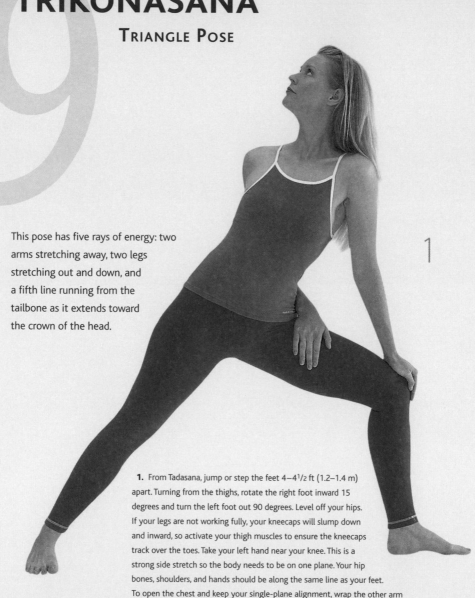

1

1. From Tadasana, jump or step the feet 4–4¹/₂ ft (1.2–1.4 m) apart. Turning from the thighs, rotate the right foot inward 15 degrees and turn the left foot out 90 degrees. Level off your hips. If your legs are not working fully, your kneecaps will slump down and inward, so activate your thigh muscles to ensure the kneecaps track over the toes. Take your left hand near your knee. This is a strong side stretch so the body needs to be on one plane. Your hip bones, shoulders, and hands should be along the same line as your feet. To open the chest and keep your single-plane alignment, wrap the other arm around the back to wedge the hand by the inner thigh, or else take hold of the back of your trousers. Assist this action by bending the front knee.

2. Draw your left sitting bone down toward your right inner heel so your hips move to the right. As you do this, straighten your left leg and slide the left hand down the leg or possibly to the floor as pictured. If you find your shoulders have come in front of your feet, and your buttocks have moved back, adjust your alignment by bringing your left hand higher up your leg. Roll your right shoulder back and enjoy the openness in the chest for several breaths before eventually releasing your right arm to vertical. Stretch out well from abdomen to feet, and from shoulders toward each hand. Intensify the line of energy from tailbone to crown of the head by sliding the shoulder blades away from the ears to keep the back of the neck long. Tuck the chin slightly in, turn the head and gaze at the right thumb.
Stay for five to ten breaths, then repeat on the right side.

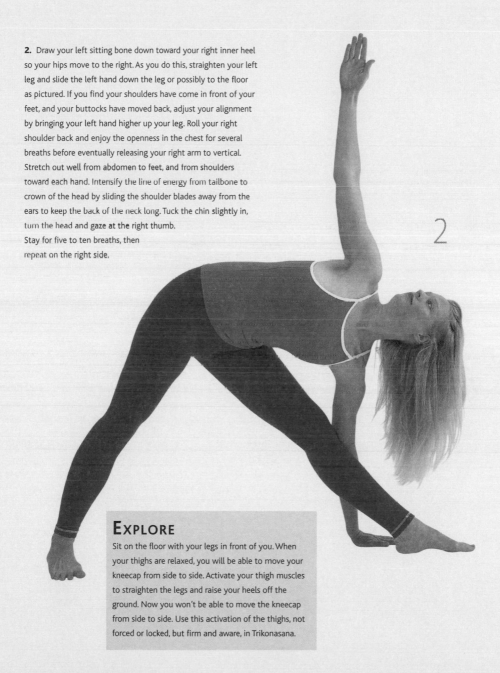

2

EXPLORE

Sit on the floor with your legs in front of you. When your thighs are relaxed, you will be able to move your kneecap from side to side. Activate your thigh muscles to straighten the legs and raise your heels off the ground. Now you won't be able to move the kneecap from side to side. Use this activation of the thighs, not forced or locked, but firm and aware, in Trikonasana.

UTTANASANA INTENSE FORWARD STRETCH

If you suffer from hypertension, keep the trunk parallel to the floor and place your hands on a chair or table. Begin working through this sequence with Roll Downs (*see* page 34).

USING A WALL

1. To maintain length in the front of the torso, practice using the wall. Stand with your feet apart and about 1 ft (30 cm) away from the wall. Lean your buttocks to the wall so your sitting bones touch it. Hold your elbows and take the arms overhead. Bend the knees and extend the torso up so the top of the breastbone moves away from the pubic bone. With knees strongly bent, reach your torso forward. Stretch as far out with the elbows as possible. Fold over your legs and let your upper body hang for ten breaths or more. With each inhalation the torso can lengthen more, and with each exhalation the crease at the top of the thighs can deepen. If you can't work in a relaxed fashion into this position, bend the knees more or walk the feet farther away from the wall. Come up on an inhalation.

2. Move away from the wall. Bring your hands onto your hips, inhale, lift your breastbone, and look up. Exhale, hinge at the hips to reach forward so the crown of the head moves in as big an arc as possible. Imagine your hip sockets and pelvis rolling forward over your thigh bones, which stay vertical.

1

2

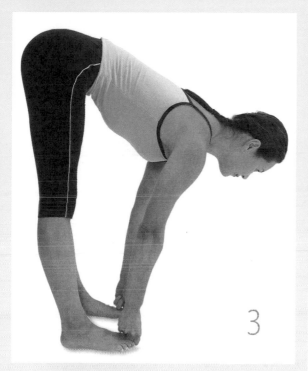

3. With your knees bent or straight, grasp your legs or ankles, or loop your big toes with finger and thumb. Increase the stretch by flattening out the back and stretching your sternum forward. Angle your sitting bones toward the sky, lengthen the back of your waist. Tilt your pelvis forward as if aiming to press your navel to your thighs—you will feel the stretch in the back of your thighs intensify.

3

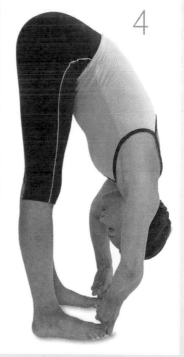

4

4. Exhale and fold forward to hold the pose. If your knees are bent, use each exhalation to work the legs straighter. If your legs are straight, firm the front thigh muscles and bring your hips forward to bring the hip joints directly over your ankles.

Check that your face is relaxed. Free the upper lip so your cheeks feel like they are dropping down toward the floor. If you have forgotten to breathe, check whether the pose is too strong for you and ease back until you free the breath.

Explore

Working the feet correctly in the standing poses helps to retrain flatfeet over time. If you have flatfeet, lift your toes up to work the arches in the standing postures. Alternatively, anchor the inner heel and mound of the big toe and, without rolling the ankles out, lift your arches like rainbows.

PAVRITTA TRIKONASANA

REVOLVED TRIANGLE POSE

This advanced pose combines balance, twisting, and forward bending. In the wide-stance poses, the farther apart the feet are, the greater the spinal extension, but the more difficult it becomes to balance.

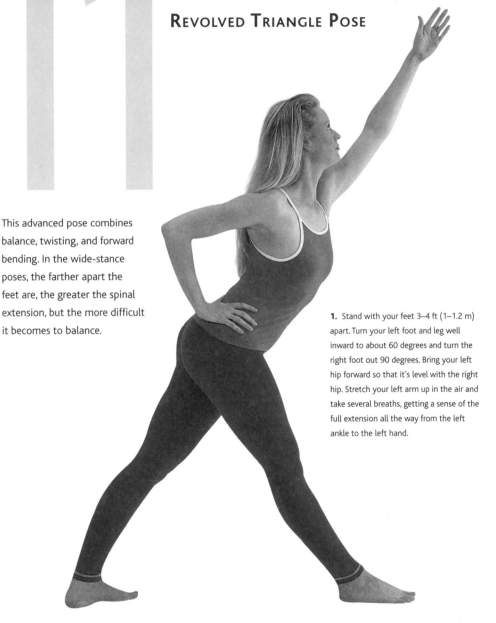

1. Stand with your feet 3–4 ft (1–1.2 m) apart. Turn your left foot and leg well inward to about 60 degrees and turn the right foot out 90 degrees. Bring your left hip forward so that it's level with the right hip. Stretch your left arm up in the air and take several breaths, getting a sense of the full extension all the way from the left ankle to the left hand.

EXPLORE

Looking down to the floor makes it easier to balance while you increase the twist in the trunk. Take several breaths gazing at the floor to allow a deeper rotation. Finally, turn the head to look forward and slowly up to the top thumb.

2. On an exhalation, reach the left arm and torso forward and down to bring the left hand to cup the floor by the right little toe. If the hand doesn't reach, place the hand on the seat of a chair or on a stack of books. With both feet and the left hand anchored, stretch the right hip back to help the extension of the spine out of the hips. Rotate the torso well to the right so the navel and heart open up to the sky. Take the right arm straight up into the air and gaze up at your right thumb.

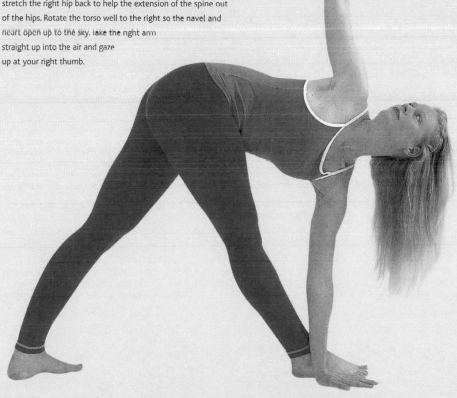

FORWARD BENDS

Sometimes in our outward-looking lives, we ignore messages from inside. Folding into ourselves quietens the mind and encourages a meditative mindset. Forward bends foster the ability to listen to the intuitive self, to the heart.

Gravity often helps us fold forward; we can go deeper into the pose by yielding rather than forcing. From the seated position, we don't even have to be concerned with balancing, and can take energy and support from the earth. The forward bends are a little like the fetal position and have nurturing qualities for when we need to feel protected.

As you fold in half from your hips, your head comes closer to your feet. The two extremes of the body come together and help you find your center. Life is full of dualities. Rather than operating from one end of the spectrum, you can find a better balance: moderation and the middle path in our world view and way of living.

By increasing pressure on the organs of the abdomen, forward bends are particularly beneficial to the digestive system. As the pelvis houses nerve ganglions of the parasympathetic nervous system, they also help balance the nervous systems. The parasympathetic nervous system directs our "rest and restore" response. Forward bends are helpful for those with active, busy (sympathetic nervous system dominant) lives, and for anyone who seeks healing and better health.

Forward bends can be done in a very active way, with strong breathing to release more deeply into the postures. Alternatively, when you are experiencing menstrual discomfort, feel fatigued, or need to revive, they can be done softly, and made more restorative using a chair or a bolster. Rest the forehead on a chair seat covered by a soft blanket. If you are more flexible, use a bolster.

Don't overdo the forward bends if you suffer from severe depression. Focus on backbends instead. Those suffering hypertension do best to keep their head above their heart. Forward bends maintain integrity of the spine, but proceed cautiously if you have back pain. If a weakness exists or if you are recovering from an injury, it is always best to build your practice in a slow and steady way. If you suffer from disk problems, that section of the spine needs to be kept concave and should not be bent forward until it is ready. Work with a teacher to incorporate forward bends into your practice bit by bit as your back strengthens. Allow 24 hours after the practice for your body to give you its feedback.

Left and oppposite:
Develop patience and
the ability to stay
longer in the
forward bends.

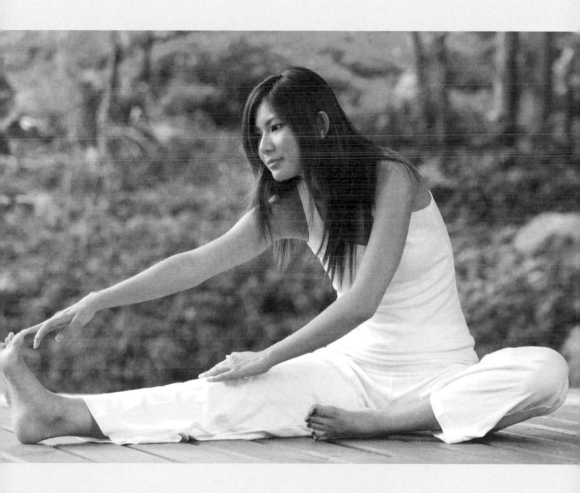

ABOUT ALIGNMENT

DISCOVERING THE ACTION OF THE PELVIS AND HIPS

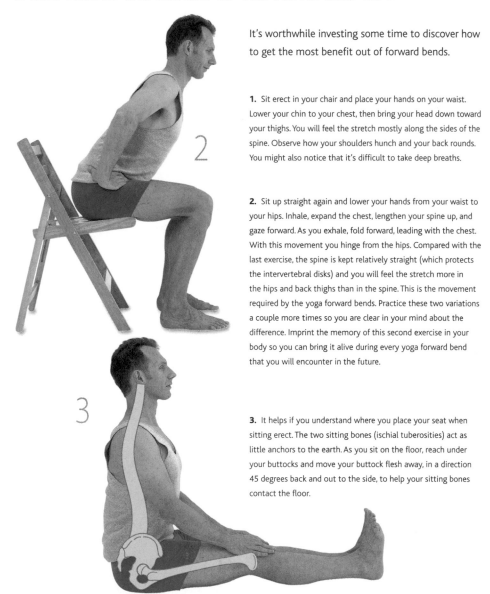

It's worthwhile investing some time to discover how to get the most benefit out of forward bends.

1. Sit erect in your chair and place your hands on your waist. Lower your chin to your chest, then bring your head down toward your thighs. You will feel the stretch mostly along the sides of the spine. Observe how your shoulders hunch and your back rounds. You might also notice that it's difficult to take deep breaths.

2. Sit up straight again and lower your hands from your waist to your hips. Inhale, expand the chest, lengthen your spine up, and gaze forward. As you exhale, fold forward, leading with the chest. With this movement you hinge from the hips. Compared with the last exercise, the spine is kept relatively straight (which protects the intervertebral disks) and you will feel the stretch more in the hips and back thighs than in the spine. This is the movement required by the yoga forward bends. Practice these two variations a couple more times so you are clear in your mind about the difference. Imprint the memory of this second exercise in your body so you can bring it alive during every yoga forward bend that you will encounter in the future.

3. It helps if you understand where you place your seat when sitting erect. The two sitting bones (ischial tuberosities) act as little anchors to the earth. As you sit on the floor, reach under your buttocks and move your buttock flesh away, in a direction 45 degrees back and out to the side, to help your sitting bones contact the floor.

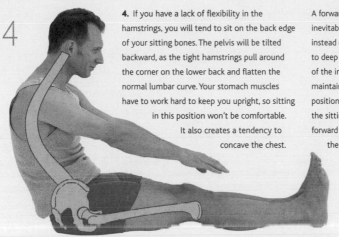

4. If you have a lack of flexibility in the hamstrings, you will tend to sit on the back edge of your sitting bones. The pelvis will be tilted backward, as the tight hamstrings pull around the corner on the lower back and flatten the normal lumbar curve. Your stomach muscles have to work hard to keep you upright, so sitting in this position won't be comfortable. It also creates a tendency to concave the chest.

A forward bend born from this position will inevitably be a forward bend from the waist, instead of the hips. Apart from closing the chest to deep breathing, by pressurizing the fronts of the intervertebral disks, the spine will not maintain a healthy alignment. The ideal starting position will be sitting right on the center of the sitting bones, so that as you fold your body forward you will roll forward to perch more on the front edge of your sitting bones.

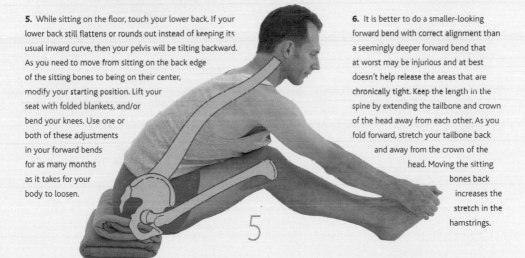

5. While sitting on the floor, touch your lower back. If your lower back still flattens or rounds out instead of keeping its usual inward curve, then your pelvis will be tilting backward. As you need to move from sitting on the back edge of the sitting bones to being on their center, modify your starting position. Lift your seat with folded blankets, and/or bend your knees. Use one or both of these adjustments in your forward bends for as many months as it takes for your body to loosen.

6. It is better to do a smaller-looking forward bend with correct alignment than a seemingly deeper forward bend that at worst may be injurious and at best doesn't help release the areas that are chronically tight. Keep the length in the spine by extending the tailbone and crown of the head away from each other. As you fold forward, stretch your tailbone back and away from the crown of the head. Moving the sitting bones back increases the stretch in the hamstrings.

7. As you fold forward, visualize your thigh bones staying still. It is actually the sockets of the hip joints that can rotate around the heads of the thigh bones to tilt the pelvis forward. When you can achieve this, the concavity in the lumbar spine will remain for the first part of the forward bend. Test this by placing your hand on your lower back to feel if you have the same curve during the first part of the forward bend. Toward the end of your stretch forward, you will feel the shape of the lumbar spine change and begin to curve outward.

8. Let go of your desire to reach your forehead to your knees. Instead, first aim the navel to the thighs. As you hinge more at the hips, your chest will come closer to your knees, and only after this will the nose come toward the shins.

DANDASANA STAFF POSE

Dandasana is the base from which we fold forward into many forward bends.

EXPLORE

Because this position is outwardly simpler than many others, it provides a good opportunity to take your attention inward. Take slow, conscious breaths. In this position it is possible to focus not only on the forward and sideward expansion of the torso, but also on the expansion of the back of the torso as you inhale and the lungs fill with air.

Sit with your legs straight out in front. If it is hard to sit with the back erect in this pose, and if you tip back, sit on one or two folded blankets. Place your fingertips or palms on the floor by the buttocks. Roll the thigh bones inward so the inner thighs come together. Have the fronts of the kneecaps and the toes pointing straight upward. Straighten the knees so the backs of the knees are stretched. Let the arms lengthen. Let the breastbone float up, but not at the cost of shortening the back. Ensure that your chin is not jutting out, but is kept parallel to the floor. Imagine your head floating on the top of your spine like a helium balloon on the top of a stick. Lighten your thoughts!

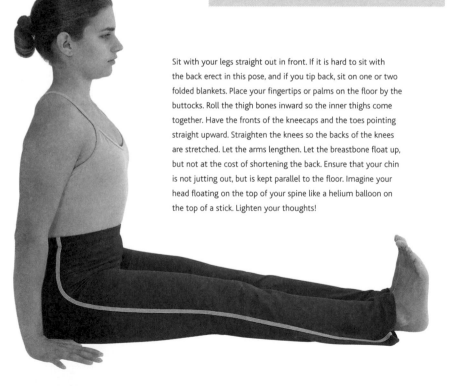

VIRASANA HERO POSE

Although children sit like this quite naturally, older, stiffer bodies can find this pose uncomfortable. Use props as necessary while you regain your flexibility.

1. Kneel on the floor with your knees together and feet wide apart. As you sit down between your feet, use your fingers to "iron" your calf muscles out to the sides and down toward the heels.

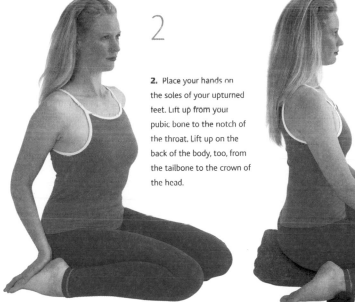

2

2. Place your hands on the soles of your upturned feet. Lift up from your pubic bone to the notch of the throat. Lift up on the back of the body, too, from the tailbone to the crown of the head.

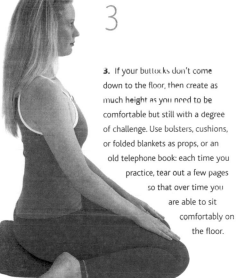

3

3. If your buttocks don't come down to the floor, then create as much height as you need to be comfortable but still with a degree of challenge. Use bolsters, cushions, or folded blankets as props, or an old telephone book: each time you practice, tear out a few pages so that over time you are able to sit comfortably on the floor.

4. If you experience knee pain, place a canvas belt or thin folded scarf deeply in the crease of the knees as they bend.

5. If this position gives pain on the tops of the feet, place some cushioning underneath the fronts of the ankles.

EXPLORE

Forward bend from this pose. Lean forward onto your hands or, if you are more flexible, stretch the arms all the way forward with fingers interlaced.

TRIANGA MUKHAIKAPADA PASCHIMOTTANASANA

THREE-LIMBED FORWARD BEND

If forward-bending Virasana is too much of a challenge for now, warm yourself up by practicing one leg at a time.

1. From Dandasana, bend your right leg back to bring the foot to the floor next to the buttocks. As in Virasana, "iron" your calf flesh out to the right. As you will tend to tilt to the left, mentally let your right sitting bone be heavy so that you stay balanced and don't tip over.

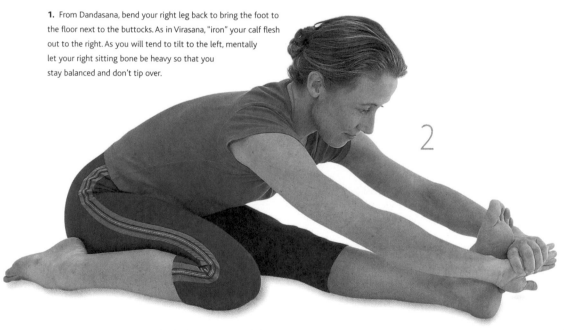

2

2. Sometimes it is useful to use a flowing movement to ease into a pose. On an inhalation, reach your arms up to the sky and then fold forward as you exhale. On the next inhalation, reach the arms out and up once more, and flow forward as you exhale. After five cycles, hold the forward bend for five to ten long breaths. Repeat on side two.

ALTERNATIVE

To align the spine and better balance the hips, place a support under one buttock.

EXPLORE

Try this way of working in some poses. If you hold a pose for 15 breaths, use the first five to adjust and deepen the posture. For the remaining ten breaths, remain steady at a still point. At this point you still the fluctuations of the body, and are moving neither from nor toward any point. Be receptive to your observations.

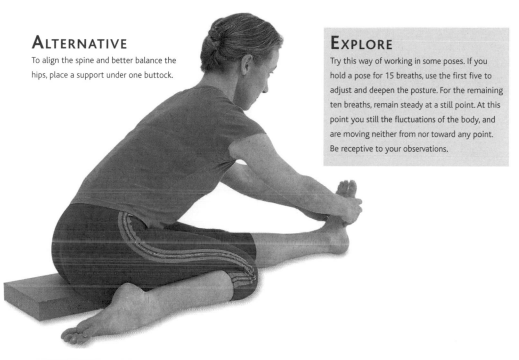

PASCHIMOTTANASANA

This is the classic Paschimottanasana. Sit in Dandasana. Keep your knees and toes pointing to the sky. Lengthen from the tailbone to the crown of the head. After several breaths "growing" the spine, inhale and raise the arms overhead, then exhale the arms and torso forward. Remember the feeling from the first exercise—keep the chest open and the breath free. Depending on your flexibility, hold one wrist around the feet, hook your toes, grasp the sides of your feet or ankles, or loop a belt around the balls of the feet. Take long, slow breaths for 10 to 15 rounds.

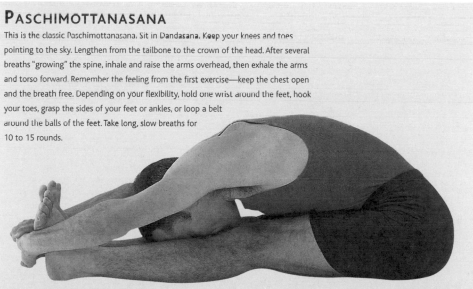

ARDHA BADDHA PADMA PASCHIMOTTANASANA

BOUND HALF-LOTUS FORWARD FOLD

Due to the position of the arms in this hip-opening stretch, it is difficult to "cheat" by rounding the shoulders. Warming up the hip will help prevent knee problems and assist the movement of the knee toward the earth. Apart from this warm-up, you can practice the ankle to knee pose (*see* page 66).

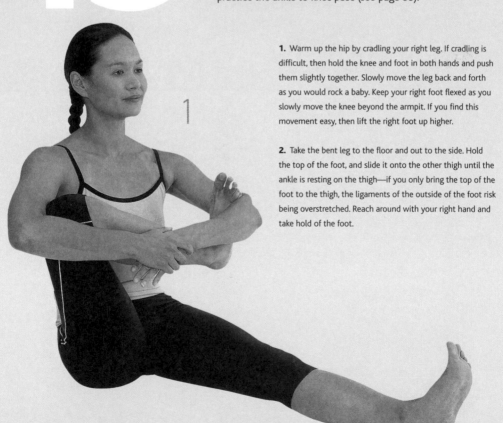

1

1. Warm up the hip by cradling your right leg. If cradling is difficult, then hold the knee and foot in both hands and push them slightly together. Slowly move the leg back and forth as you would rock a baby. Keep your right foot flexed as you slowly move the knee beyond the armpit. If you find this movement easy, then lift the right foot up higher.

2. Take the bent leg to the floor and out to the side. Hold the top of the foot, and slide it onto the other thigh until the ankle is resting on the thigh—if you only bring the top of the foot to the thigh, the ligaments of the outside of the foot risk being overstretched. Reach around with your right hand and take hold of the foot.

3

3. Stretch forward and take your right hand to the right foot, ankle or shin. Release your left knee down to the floor. Hold for five to ten breaths. Repeat on the other side.

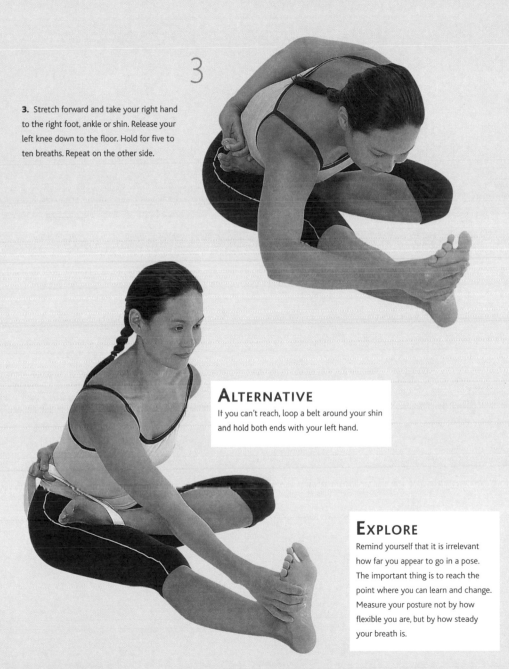

ALTERNATIVE

If you can't reach, loop a belt around your shin and hold both ends with your left hand.

EXPLORE

Remind yourself that it is irrelevant how far you appear to go in a pose. The important thing is to reach the point where you can learn and change. Measure your posture not by how flexible you are, but by how steady your breath is.

UPAVISTA KONASANA

SEATED WIDE-ANGLE POSE SEQUENCE

16

Have patience as you hold this pose.
Wait for the body to let you in.

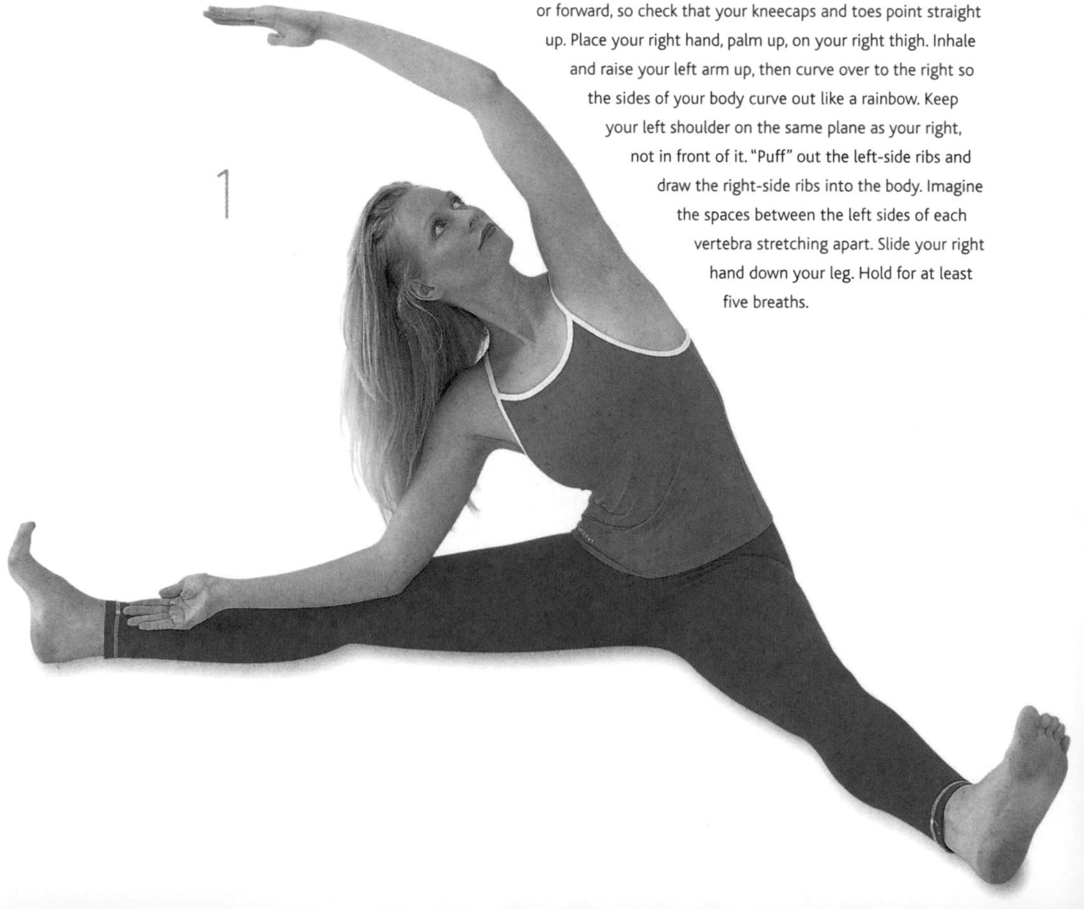

1. Sit with your legs out to the sides at about a 90-degree angle. In this pose it is easy to let the kneecaps roll backward or forward, so check that your kneecaps and toes point straight up. Place your right hand, palm up, on your right thigh. Inhale and raise your left arm up, then curve over to the right so the sides of your body curve out like a rainbow. Keep your left shoulder on the same plane as your right, not in front of it. "Puff" out the left-side ribs and draw the right-side ribs into the body. Imagine the spaces between the left sides of each vertebra stretching apart. Slide your right hand down your leg. Hold for at least five breaths.

1

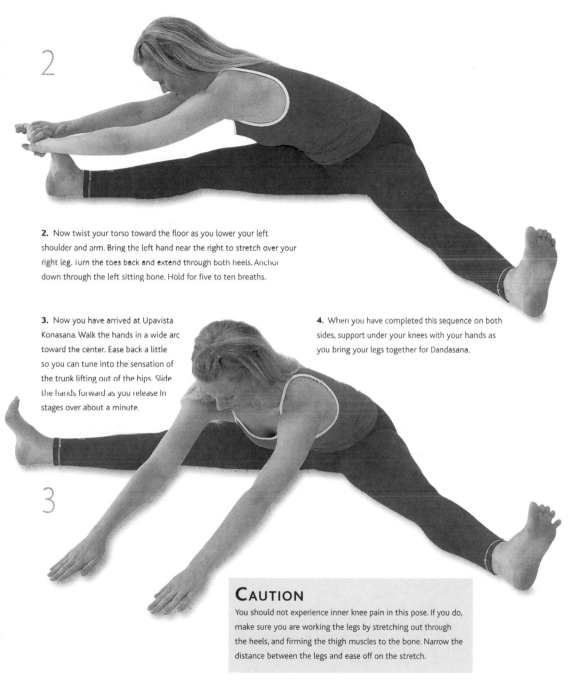

2

2. Now twist your torso toward the floor as you lower your left shoulder and arm. Bring the left hand near the right to stretch over your right leg. Turn the toes back and extend through both heels. Anchor down through the left sitting bone. Hold for five to ten breaths.

3. Now you have arrived at Upavista Konasana. Walk the hands in a wide arc toward the center. Ease back a little so you can tune into the sensation of the trunk lifting out of the hips. Slide the hands forward as you release in stages over about a minute.

4. When you have completed this sequence on both sides, support under your knees with your hands as you bring your legs together for Dandasana.

3

CAUTION

You should not experience inner knee pain in this pose. If you do, make sure you are working the legs by stretching out through the heels, and firming the thigh muscles to the bone. Narrow the distance between the legs and ease off on the stretch.

BADDHA KONASANA

COBBLER'S POSE

Translated from Sanskrit as "Bound Angle Pose," this position is also called "Cobbler's Pose" because it is the position in which shoemakers in India sit to work.

1. Raise your seat with a support such as a cushion and bring the soles of your feet together. Draw your heels up close toward you. Use the pressure of your hands on the floor behind you to tilt the pelvis forward. As you do so, let the breastbone float up. These two movements will begin the opening along the inner thighs and groin. With the support of your hands behind you, move the knees away from each other, back and down to the floor. If your hips are tight, this may be as far as you go in this pose for today.

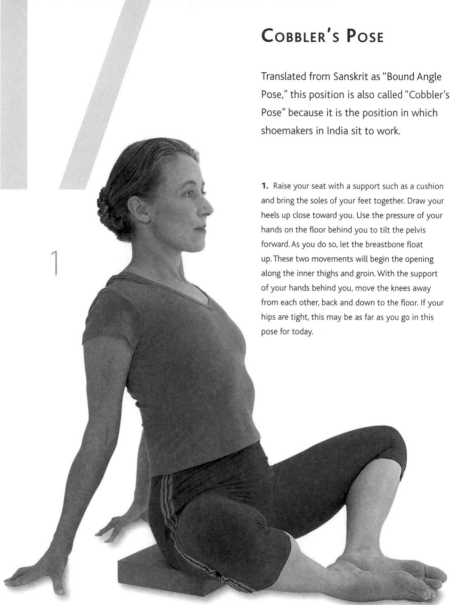

2

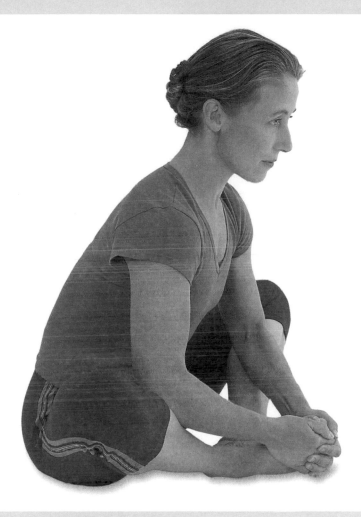

2. If your pelvis tips forward easily, you can dispense with the cushion before bending your elbows into the calves and binding the feet with your hands. Inhale and create the sensation of the torso lifting out of the pelvis. Exhale and deepen the fold. On each inhalation, lengthen from pubic bone to throat; each exhalation is an opportunity to move out and down. Rather than butterflying the knees up and down, work with the breath to soften the tight areas. Breathe evenly for five to ten rounds.

EXPLORE

Sit on the floor in this position whenever possible. Lean back against the sofa in Cobbler's Pose while you watch television.

SUPTA PADANGUSTASANA

RECLINING BIG TOE POSE

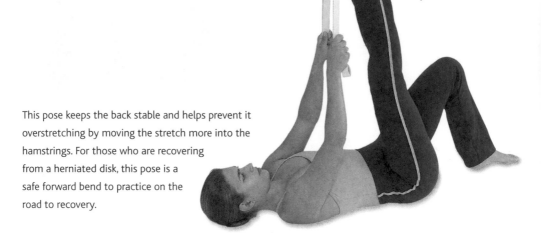

This pose keeps the back stable and helps prevent it overstretching by moving the stretch more into the hamstrings. For those who are recovering from a herniated disk, this pose is a safe forward bend to practice on the road to recovery.

1. Lie on your back with your knees bent up. Lift your right leg and loop a belt around the ball of the foot. Straighten the leg. As you inhale, imagine a line of energy extending from right buttock to right heel. As you exhale, yield a little to stretch the back of the leg more.

2. Release tension in the shoulders. Check the chin is not jutting up in the air—if it is, slide the back of the head away to bring it down.

3. If you are ready to move on to stage two, straighten the left leg along the floor and stretch out through both heels. As your flexibility grows, your leg will form an acute angle with your torso. Then you will be able to work the pose by holding the big toe of the raised foot. Until this comes, use the belt. After one to two minutes in this position, inhale and curl your head and upper back off the floor to bring your nose to your knee. Walk your hands higher up the belt. Hold for seven breaths and when you exhale down, keep the hands at that height and, seemingly miraculously, your body may be able to accept the increased stretch.

4. For this next stage, it is important to keep the left leg straight as it acts as your anchor. In the beginning, use your left hand to press down on the top of your left thigh. Holding the belt or side of your foot, take your right leg out to the side. Although you may not get that high during this practice, aim to take your toes to the floor at shoulder level. Do this movement slowly so you don't lose the grounding force of the left upper thigh and left heel. If you start to tip, come back up and press both sides of the sacrum down to the floor before lowering again.

Hold for five to ten breaths.

4

5

5. Come back to center and hold your big toe, or both ends of the belt, in your left hand. Turn your toes inward and anchor down the sacrum on the right side. It helps to press down with your thumb at the root of the thigh. Take the leg over to the left and hold for five to ten breaths. Come back to stretching through the center before lowering the leg down to repeat on the second side.

EXPLORE

Before you do this hip-releasing sequence, lie flat and look at your feet. Your toes will be turned out—measure how much the toes of each foot are turned out, checking the difference between sides. This sequence releases the hips. Visually measure it again after each side.

GOMUKHASANA COW FACE POSE

Sometimes the poses we find most difficult are the very ones we can benefit most from practicing.

EXPLORE

If this pose comes easily to you, lower the arms and lean forward onto the hands. Then try bringing your heels forward so they are on the same transverse plane as your buttocks. Now place your hands on the floor in front of you and lean forward to deepen the stretch.

1. Warm the hips up first by sitting cross-legged. Take the left ankle and place it on the top of the right knee. Make sure it is the ankle, not the outer part of the top of the foot, so that the ligaments in that area are not stretched too much. If your top shin is more or less parallel to the floor, then you can place your hands on the floor in front and stretch forward. Otherwise, breathe into the hips from an upright position to help loosen them. Repeat on the other side. Another useful warm-up is cradling the leg (see page 58).

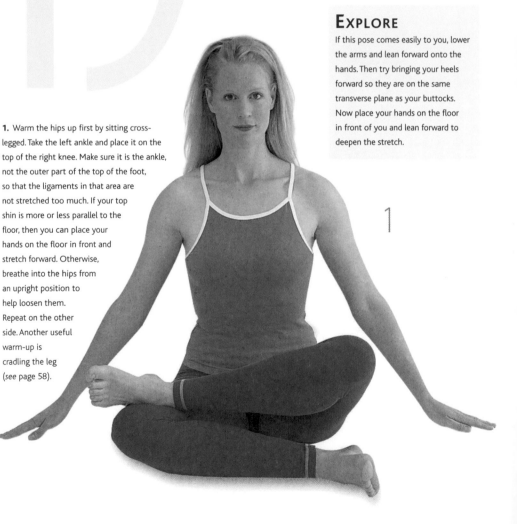

1

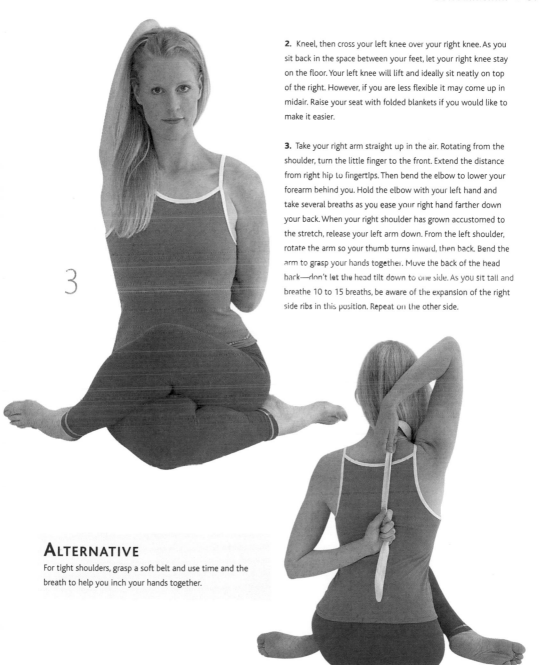

2. Kneel, then cross your left knee over your right knee. As you sit back in the space between your feet, let your right knee stay on the floor. Your left knee will lift and ideally sit neatly on top of the right. However, if you are less flexible it may come up in midair. Raise your seat with folded blankets if you would like to make it easier.

3. Take your right arm straight up in the air. Rotating from the shoulder, turn the little finger to the front. Extend the distance from right hip to fingertips. Then bend the elbow to lower your forearm behind you. Hold the elbow with your left hand and take several breaths as you ease your right hand farther down your back. When your right shoulder has grown accustomed to the stretch, release your left arm down. From the left shoulder, rotate the arm so your thumb turns inward, then back. Bend the arm to grasp your hands together. Move the back of the head back—don't let the head tilt down to one side. As you sit tall and breathe 10 to 15 breaths, be aware of the expansion of the right side ribs in this position. Repeat on the other side.

ALTERNATIVE

For tight shoulders, grasp a soft belt and use time and the breath to help you inch your hands together.

AFTER FORWARD FOLDING

20

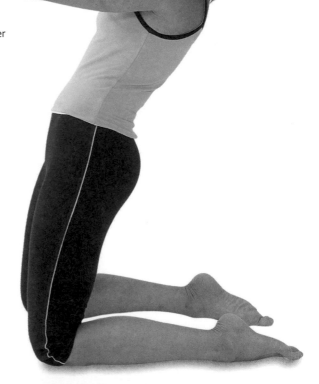

These stretches act as counterposes after some intense forward bending.

Z POSE

Kneel on a cushioned surface if you like. Stretch the arms forward, parallel to the floor. Tuck the tailbone under, open the groin and lean back to form a "Z" shape.

SAVASANA VARIATION
Corpse Pose Variation
Resting in Corpse Pose with the arms overhead
brings a slight backbend to balance the body.

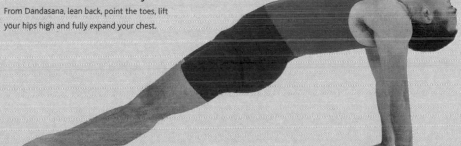

PURVOTTANASANA
Stretch on the East Side of the Body
From Dandasana, lean back, point the toes, lift
your hips high and fully expand your chest.

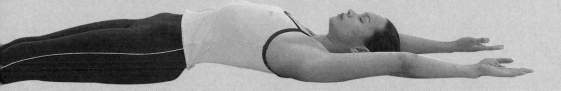

PURVOTTANASANA
Easier Version
Begin with bent knees, lift the
hips and chest up, then
stretch the chin away.

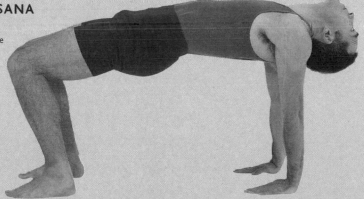

BACKBENDS

Like the forward bends, the backbends help keep the spine supple and well aligned to promote good functioning of the nerves, which innervate the rest of the body.

BACKBENDS

Sit erect, take a deep inhalation, look up and notice how the spine seems to lengthen, grow and extend. Congratulations! You have begun a lovely backbend!

If you think of what you do every day, you will notice that many of your activities involve bending forward. Sitting at a desk to work, at a table to eat, driving, cleaning house, or gardening all tend to shorten the front of the body. Even the habit of looking at the ground while walking can put a stoop in good posture. Backbends realign the spine, counteract rounded shoulders, and help us move with poise and grace.

Backbends are exciting, energy-raising, and warming. Repeat any active backbend a few times in a cold room and you will soon feel the heat created. Backbends keep the spine young and supple. They activate the abdominal region and stimulate blood supply to the kidneys, reproductive system, and digestive organs.

The vertebral column houses the main subtle energy pathway, the Sushumna Nadi. Backbends help shunt energy up the spine and through the chakras—the centers of energy—along the way. Working especially from the second to fifth chakras, energy blockages are released and stagnant areas invigorated.

You need courage, determination, and willpower to hold strong backbends, the very same qualities that are linked to the third chakra at the solar plexus. Backbends build character, strength, and confidence, which is what people mean when they refer to someone who "has backbone." You can develop "backbone" to deal with change and pressure in other parts of your life as you explore your full range of flexibility. Integrity of the spine can help create integrity of the mind. It is hard to think about anything else when you are breathing strongly in a strong backbend, so, by making the mind and body alert, backbends help combat depression and lethargy.

When we feel unsafe we instinctively fold in on ourselves. Bending backward counteracts this curling up and brings us out of our shelter. Lengthening and opening along the belly exposes our visceral organs, giving us practice in dealing with vulnerability. Backbends are like exploring uncharted territory. They allow us to practice spreading awareness to unfamiliar parts of the body. We never see our backs directly, needing instead to twist around to catch a reflection in a mirror. Bending backward is leaning into new terrain, requiring us to conquer the fear of the unknown.

In opening the heart center, backbends are enormously uplifting. The chest lifts and widens to encourage better breathing and full expansion of the lungs. Expanding the heart center uncramps, rejuvenates, and welcomes joyful vitality into your life.

Always warm up with some standing postures before beginning backbends. To really feel your backbends develop, repeat the pose three times. The body does tend to feel the effects of holding backbends, so follow with some of the counterposes on pages 84–85.

Those suffering from hypertension or heart trouble should work with an experienced teacher. Avoid strong backbends during menstruation, pregnancy, and for eight weeks after giving birth. Those with a herniated disk, lumbar injury, peptic or duodenal hernia, or who have recently had surgery can practice mild backbends. If weakness of the back or discomfort is present, build up your practice slowly and progressively.

Above and opposite: You must protect the vulnerable lower back and neck, making these parts stronger and bringing awareness to them.

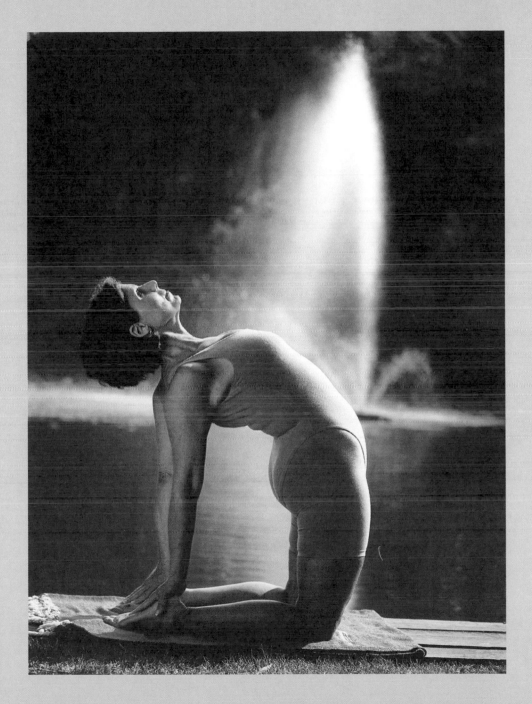

ABOUT ALIGNMENT

SPECIAL PREPARATIONS FOR BETTER BACKBENDS

Stretch the legs and trunk and open the shoulders before backbending.
Warm up the body with these exercises and your backbending will
come more easily.

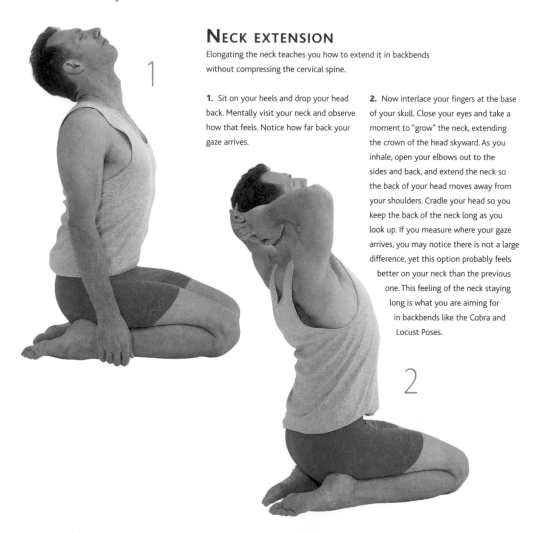

NECK EXTENSION

Elongating the neck teaches you how to extend it in backbends
without compressing the cervical spine.

1. Sit on your heels and drop your head
back. Mentally visit your neck and observe
how that feels. Notice how far back your
gaze arrives.

2. Now interlace your fingers at the base
of your skull. Close your eyes and take a
moment to "grow" the neck, extending
the crown of the head skyward. As you
inhale, open your elbows out to the
sides and back, and extend the neck so
the back of your head moves away from
your shoulders. Cradle your head so you
keep the back of the neck long as you
look up. If you measure where your gaze
arrives, you may notice there is not a large
difference, yet this option probably feels
better on your neck than the previous
one. This feeling of the neck staying
long is what you are aiming for
in backbends like the Cobra and
Locust Poses.

SHOULDER EXTENSION

These shoulder exercises give more lift with "longer" released arms.

1. Stand side-on to the wall, at a distance of about 10 in (25 cm). The more flexible you are, the closer you will get to the wall. Stretch the arm nearer to the wall as high up as you can reach, touching your palm to the wall. Take several slow breaths, feeling as if you are hanging down from the raised hand. Now take it back 45 degrees (pictured) for another ten or so breaths. Finally, take it farther behind, to be, if possible, parallel to the floor. Lean your chest forward and breathe. After doing one side, if you relax your arms and then swing them together to join the palms you might find the worked arm "longer" than the other. Repeat on the other side.

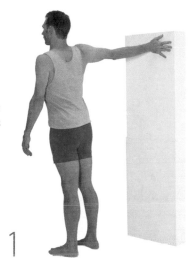

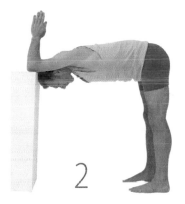

2. Bring your elbows to the padded edge of a table so they are shoulder-width apart. Step back so your ankles are under your hips and you form a table shape. Bring your palms together and lower the head, if possible, so the neck is in line with the spine. You will feel a stretch in the shoulders. This is table prayer pose. As you hold the position, let the side ribs soften down. After ten breaths here, slowly lower your hands between your shoulder blades so your fingers point toward your tailbone. Move slowly between these two positions a few times. To come up, walk in, lift your head and scoop up.

SUPTA VIRASANA Reclining Hero Pose

The iliopsoas is a deep muscle running from the inner thigh bone to the lumbar vertebrae. When this muscle is tight or contracted, it pulls us into a forward bend. A released iliopsoas muscle is essential for healthy backbending. Begin in Virasana (see page 55). Lean back on your elbows, then come up a little so you can lift your pubic bone up as you stretch your tailbone away. Breathe here for a while. Maintaining the tilt of the pelvis, keep your floating ribs from jutting out as you lower your buttocks to the floor. Gaze straight ahead or take the head back and stretch the chin away. If this stretch is too strong on the thighs, practice the lunge outlined in the first part of Anjaneyasana (see page 74), and Virabhadrasana I (see page 40).

ANJANEYASANA CRESCENT MOON POSE

The iliopsoas-lengthening lunge part of this pose is a good warm-up for all the other backbends. There are two directions of movement of energy in this pose. The movement from the back of the waist down extends through the back foot and allows the hips to descend. The upward stretch beginning at the waist radiates energy upward.

1. Kneel on a cushioned surface and step your left leg forward. Cup the floor with your fingertips and bring the hips forward to lunge. Ground through the back knee as you allow time and the breath to farther open the left groin and lower the hips. Give the muscles time to relax in this pose. When you have connected to the grounding force of gravity and the hips have got the message to drop, lower the chest slightly, lengthen forward with the breastbone, press the fingertips to the floor and lift up to increase the bend in the back. Then practice on the other side.

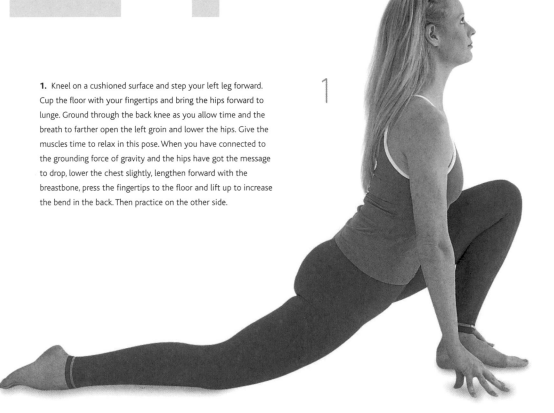

1

2. Return to lunge on the first side. When you have followed the same steps, bring your hands to your front knee. Then reach the arms forward and cross the fingers for strength. Lift the upper body up to the sky. Imagine someone is gently pulling you by your wrists up out of your hips. At the same time, release the hips so they sink more to the floor. If the pressure of your back knee against the floor is uncomfortable, press down more through the top of the back foot. If you are comfortable and feel you have a good lifting sensation, proceed to the next step.

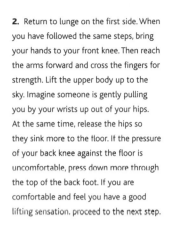

2

EXPLORE

The thoracic region bends back less easily than the lumbar and cervical regions. Remain aware of where you are working from when practicing backbends. Otherwise you will be at risk of overworking the lower back and neck and underworking the mid and upper back. Extend and arch the whole spine evenly to avoid compressing the spaces between the vertebrae.

3. Lengthen the spine farther, then lift the breastbone up, curve the back backward, and bring the shoulders and arms back. Drop the head back and stretch the chin away. Inhale to come out of the pose and repeat with the right leg forward.

3

USTRASANA Camel Pose

Forming the camel's hump strongly stretches the thighs, opens the groin, and lifts the heart. The fifth chakra at the throat is activated in this posture where the head is tilted back and the chin stretched away.

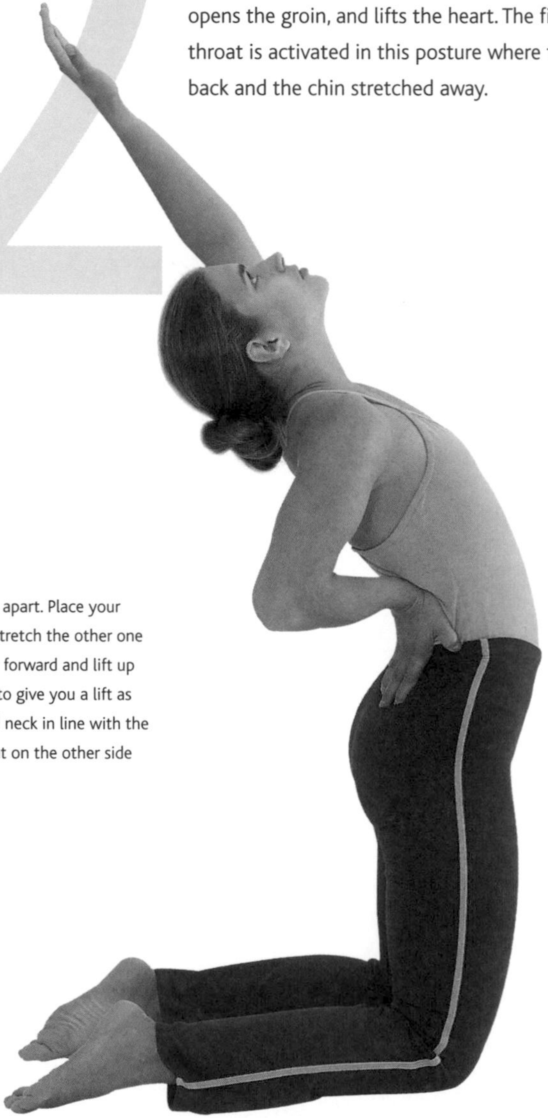

22

1. Kneel with your knees hip-width apart. Place your right hand on your lower back and stretch the other one straight up in the air. Push your hips forward and lift up the breastbone. Use the raised arm to give you a lift as you extend back. Keep the head and neck in line with the upper arm and breathe freely. Repeat on the other side before sitting down on the heels.

1

2. While kneeling, tuck your toes under. This time, lift up well through the top arm and bring the other arm down so your fingers hold the heel. Don't twist the body. Keep both hips and front ribs facing forward. After five breaths, repeat on the second side.

3. Now you are warmed up for the full Ustrasana. From kneeling, take both hands to the small of your back and massage it a little. The energy moves down from the back of the waist to ground through the knees. Remember the feeling of lift that the raised arms gave to the first two exercises. Maintain the lift through the spine from the back of the waist upward to open the chest. Take the hands one by one to the heels. Then use them as your anchor to open the groin and stretch the hips forward, aiming to have the thigh bones vertical. Continue to lift the breastbone to the sky as you roll your shoulders back. Finally, take your head back. When it is time to come up, pressurize your feet on the floor, inhale and come up. After three repetitions, release the back by using Balasana or Child Pose (see page 23).

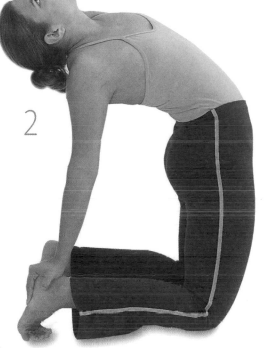

2

3

EXPLORE

You can increase the challenge of this pose by untucking the toes so that the tops of the feet are on the floor. To further deepen the pose, bring the knees and feet together. Remember that both the front and back sides of the body must participate equally in the backbends. Exhale and soften the face to release tension.

23 SETU BANDHASANA BRIDGE POSE

Strengthen your body and expand your heart center in this pose.

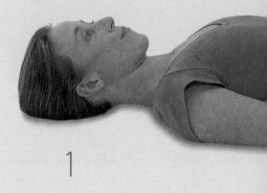

1. Lie on your back with your knees bent. Have your knees and feet body-width apart. Lift your pelvis slightly so your buttocks just begin to move off the floor. As you take several breaths in this position, lengthen your tailbone toward your feet. Now peel your vertebrae, one by one, off the floor. Tuck the shoulders under, one by one, and move the breastbone toward the chin.

2. While the breastbone moves toward your chin, the tailbone moves toward the knees and the knees stretch away from you. Don't let your knees splay apart—keep them only as wide as your hips by squeezing the inner thighs toward one another. Check that excess tension is not building up in the neck. After holding for five to ten breaths, come down and rest. Repeat twice more. Then hug the knees into the chest and rock from side to side to release the back.

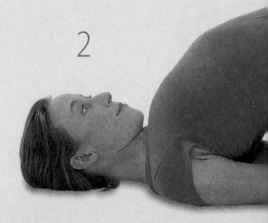

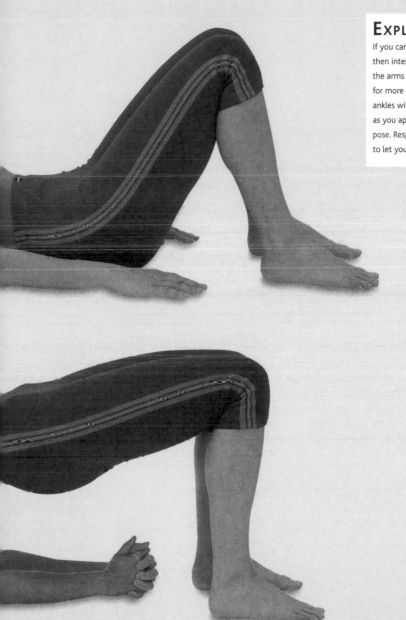

EXPLORE

If you can straighten your elbows, then interlace the fingers and press the arms down. If your body is ready for more of a challenge, grasp your ankles with your hands. Have patience as you approach each new edge in a pose. Respect the body and wait for it to let you in.

MATSYASANA FISH POSE

24

Matsyasana is a good pose for releasing the neck after practicing Shoulderstand (*see* page 112), Plough Pose (*see* page 116), and Knee to Ear Pose (*see* page 117).

1. Sit on the floor with your legs in front. For this whole sequence you need to press the insides of the feet and thighs together. Lean back on your hands and pressurize the palms to the floor. Lengthen the arms and lift up with the chest. Fully engage your mind in this process. Take your head back and don't forget to breathe. Lift the head and inhale as you come up out of the pose.

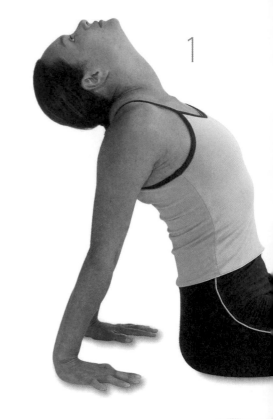

1

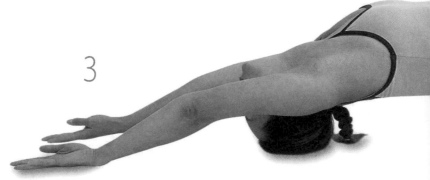

3

2. If you would like to take it a step farther, lean back on your elbows so your fingers are by your buttocks. Press down into the elbows and lift the chest into a beautiful arch. With each inhalation, feel the spine move into the core of the body and elongate, setting it up for you to deepen the pose on the exhalation.

3. From position 2, slide your elbows apart to lower down on the crown of your head. Stretch your arms overhead, and reach the fingers away actively. To release, bring the arms to your sides, inhale to lift the head slightly, and then slide it away and lie flat.

EXPLORE

Bring your mental sensitivity to the back of the body; feel how it stretches and the skin thins out.

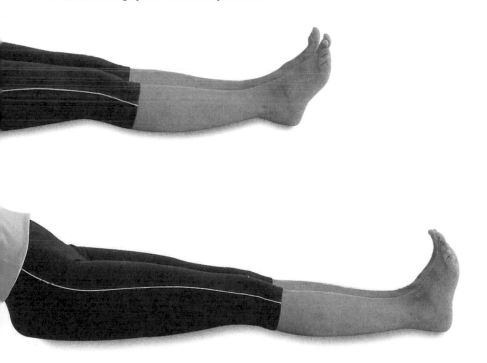

URDVA DHANURASANA

UPWARD-FACING BOW POSE

Many people who have difficulty rising into this pose assume that it is because they lack strength, but often it is due to a lack of shoulder flexibility. If your shoulders are tight, then first practice releasing the shoulders with the table prayer pose from the section on alignment (*see* Shoulder Extension 2 on page 73). Prepare for this demanding pose with Crescent Moon Pose (*see* page 74) to open the groin and stretch the thighs.

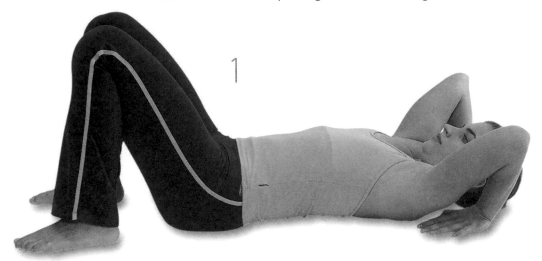

1

1. Lie on your back, with your knees bent. The action on the back is better when the feet are not turned out, so check that your toes are pointing forward. Place your palms near the shoulders, fingers pointing in the direction of the hips. Hold here as you allow the anchoring of the heels to earth to take place. Fully feeling the weight of the heels, slowly peel the back up off the floor and lift the hips. Let the grounding of the body come through the heels, then down into the earth.

CAUTION

This pose is not advisable in cases of slipped disk, hernia, heart problems and high blood pressure, during menstruation, pregnancy, or in the postnatal period.

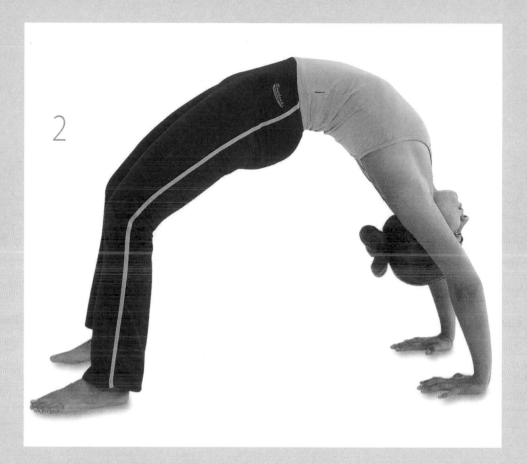

2

2. Watching the breath, wait for the inner cue to move. Catch it when it comes by lifting your hips as you pressurize the palms and straighten the arms to lift your body into the full position.

3. Now that you are up, adjust your feet, which may have turned out. Press your inner thighs closer together. As in Bridge Pose (*see* page 78), push the groin up. Let the spine move in toward the front of the body while you consolidate the pose, then expand it in both directions away from the back of the waist. It might help to lengthen toward the tailbone if you lift your heels off the ground for a few breaths.

EXPLORE

Your yoga practice is not just how you look in a pose. It is how you are when you are not in it, too. This includes going into and coming out of a pose. Never collapse out of a pose, but maintain a steady control. When resting in between repetitions, take your awareness to the back of the body (including the back of the brain) and you will recover more quickly.

AFTER BACKBENDING

Always practice a couple of twists and forward bends after a session on backbending.

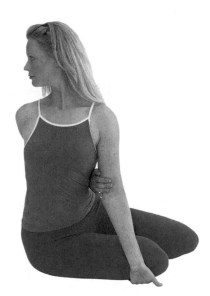

ROCKING

Your back will enjoy this massage. Lying down, hug your knees into your chest and rock slowly from side to side. Then press your knees away, resisting with your arms. More of your lower back will come into contact with the floor as you rock.

BHARADVAJASANA Sage Twist 1

Spiraling outward and upward releases tension from the whole torso.

PASSIVE OPENING OUT TWIST

Stretching out like a starfish expands the heart.

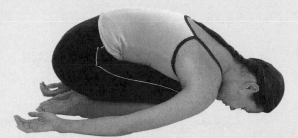

BALASANA CHILD POSE

This relaxing pose cultivates the sense of release and surrender.

YOGAMUDRASANA Sealing Pose

This pose quietens the mind and is very comfortable.

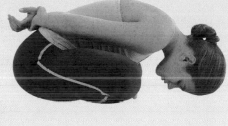

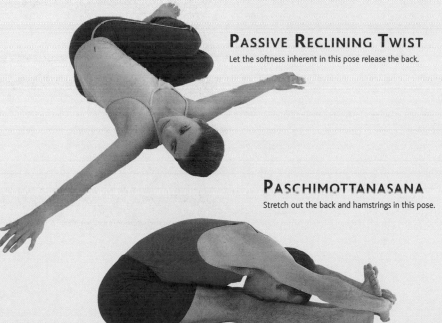

PASSIVE RECLINING TWIST

Let the softness inherent in this pose release the back.

PASCHIMOTTANASANA

Stretch out the back and hamstrings in this pose.

TWISTS

From where you're sitting, twist around to one side for ten breaths. Wind yourself up tight. Coil around with every cell in your torso. Now uncoil. Feel different? A twist is a great opportunity to turn and see things from a different angle.

When you feel wound up by life, temporarily increase the winding with a twist. Spiral up to the sky, then feel the tension dissipate as you undo and consciously unwind out of the twist.

The vertebrae are held in place by many small muscles and ligaments that need to be exercised to stay in top shape. Should they weaken, or should the distribution of strength through the back be uneven, the spine can be pulled out of alignment. A decrease of innervation can cause all sorts of problems in other areas and body systems.

An often used analogy is that of the dish sponge. When the sponge is full of soapy water, it can be squeezed out, ready to fill with clean water. That's what twists do to the abdominal organs. They temporarily increase the pressure on them so that the deoxygenated blood is squeezed out. Then the organs receive fresh oxygen and nutrient-rich blood.

Our well-being depends on a happy spine. Twists prevent stiffness of the spine and counteract any decrease in mobility that makes one look and feel old. Wringing out the body releases lots of built-up tension. Twists can reduce headaches and stiffness in the neck and shoulders. Depending on the cause, they can work miracles in relieving backache, as they stretch and strengthen the tiny muscles that link each vertebra to its neighbor. They help the spine maintain a healthy alignment.

Twists nourish the disks between the vertebrae. As the intervertebral disks have no direct blood supply from adulthood on, the bending forward, backward, and twisting of yoga postures brings them the nutrients they need to keep healthy. When practicing twists, take some time to lengthen the torso first to be sure you are elongating, not compressing the spine.

Twists increase vitality and energy and boost the flow of prana around the body. By placing pressure on the organs of digestion, then releasing it, twists feed the digestive fire. Through their massaging effect on the organs, they eliminate sluggishness and ward off constipation.

Don't practice twists intensively if you have a hernia or have had recent surgery; consult an experienced teacher first. Proceed with extreme caution if you have disk problems, as the twists will need to be implemented gradually, allowing for any delayed feedback from your body. Women benefit from practicing twists between periods to relieve menstrual cramps. During menstruation, use gentle twists. In pregnancy, practice simple twists in an open way (for example, without compressing the abdomen against the thigh) and flow in and out of them a few times without holding for long.

Above and opposite: A twist offers a mental break and a time to view things from a fresh perspective.

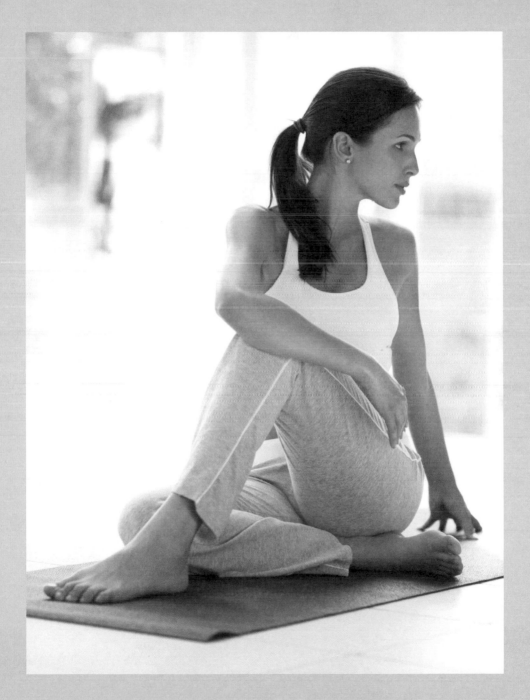

BHARADVAJASANA I

SAGE TWIST I

Spiraling outward and upward releases
tension from the whole torso.

1. From Dandasana (*see* page 54), bring
your legs around to the left and tuck the
right foot under the left ankle. Have both
knees facing forward. Hold your right knee
with your left hand. Bring your right hand
to the floor behind you. Sink the sitting
bones toward the floor, and take as many
breaths as you need to extend up from
your base. If this starting position is not
at all comfortable for you, place a small
support, like a cushion or folded blanket,
under one buttock to level yourself off.

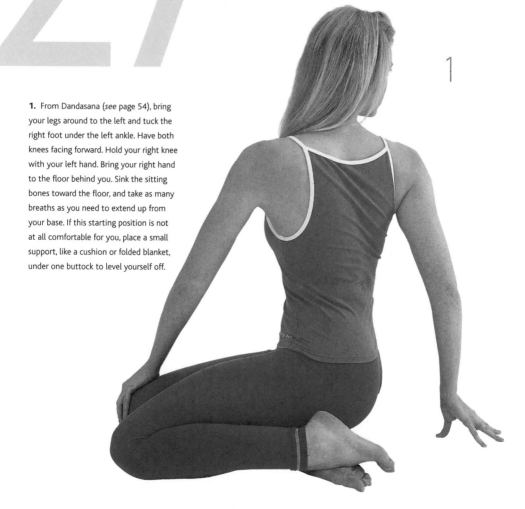

1

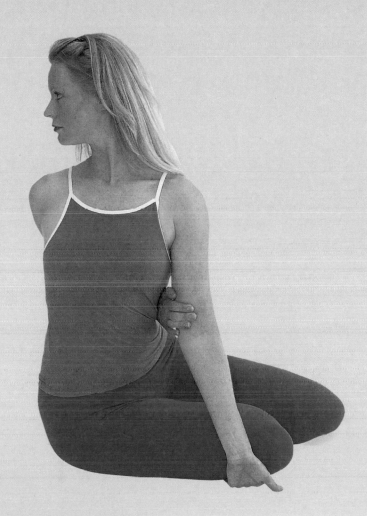

2

2. When you have lengthened well, revolving from the hips, spiral into the fuller twist, moving with the support of your abdominal organs. If possible, slide your left hand under the knee, wrist facing out. Catch hold of your left arm with your right hand and look back over your shoulder. More advanced practitioners can anchor down well through the left sitting bone, allowing the shortened left side of the waist to elongate as the right naturally does. After five to ten breaths, sit on your heels to rest and feel the effects, before repeating on side two.

EXPLORE

Bring your head into the pose just as you would normally. Measure with your eyes how far around you go. Now turn just your neck and head back to the front. This time, close your eyes and, with awareness, bring your neck and head back around into the twist. Go only as far as feels healthily comfortable for your neck. Open your eyes and note how far you reached.

JATHARA PARIVARTANASANA

REVOLVED ABDOMEN POSE

Weak abdominal muscles often contribute to chronic back pain. This exercise, practiced daily, will quickly strengthen the muscles. The passive reclining twist is less strengthening, but wonderful for easing pain caused by tight back muscles pulling on the vertebrae and causing nerve irritation and pain.

Passive Reclining Twist

1. Lie on your back with your knees bent up close to the chest. Take your arms out to the sides. Keep your knees in close to the body and slowly drop both your knees over to the right side, aiming them toward your elbow. Relax both knees and feet down to the floor. If your knees or feet don't arrive there, rest them on a folded blanket. Turn your head to the left side. There is nothing more to do in this pose. Bring your attention to actively undoing the parts of the body that are holding on to tension. Check the buttocks, back, shoulders, and face. Stay in this pose for one to two minutes. To come up, turn your head back to center first, lift the top leg in the air, then the other leg, then proceed to side two.

EXPLORE

You can move the emphasis of the passive twist up and down the back depending on where you place your knees. If your thighs are more at right angles with the torso, the emphasis of the twist is farther down the back. If your knees start close to your chest and land close to your elbow, the twist moves up the back.

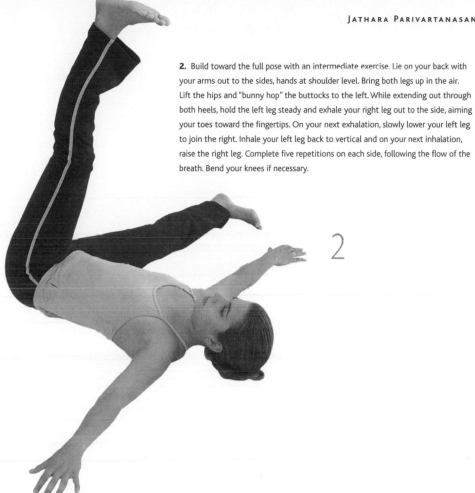

2. Build toward the full pose with an intermediate exercise. Lie on your back with your arms out to the sides, hands at shoulder level. Bring both legs up in the air. Lift the hips and "bunny hop" the buttocks to the left. While extending out through both heels, hold the left leg steady and exhale your right leg out to the side, aiming your toes toward the fingertips. On your next exhalation, slowly lower your left leg to join the right. Inhale your left leg back to vertical and on your next inhalation, raise the right leg. Complete five repetitions on each side, following the flow of the breath. Bend your knees if necessary.

3. If your legs can come to at least a 90-degree angle, then you are ready for the full pose with straight legs. If, when you raise your legs in the air, they don't come at least to vertical, keep your knees bent as you follow these instructions. "Bunny hop" your buttocks 6 in (15 cm) to the left, so that your toes angle off toward the right hand. Exhale to lower both legs to the right at the same time. If you can, catch hold of the feet. Your top heel will usually sit behind the other. To increase the twist, reach the top heel away as you "revolve" your abdominal muscles in the opposite direction. Anchor as much of the left side of your trunk and left shoulder to the floor as you can. Turn your head to gaze at your left hand. Do an even number of repetitions on each side, exhaling down and inhaling up. For the final repetition, stay in this twist for five breaths before inhaling up.

PASSIVE OPENING OUT TWIST

29

Stretching out like a starfish expands the heart.
Open yourself to a childlike feeling of happiness.

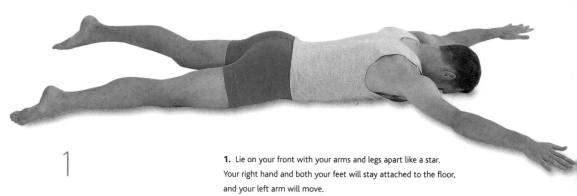

1

1. Lie on your front with your arms and legs apart like a star.
Your right hand and both your feet will stay attached to the floor,
and your left arm will move.

EXPLORE

In this position, one lung is more open than the other. Explore
the expansion of the side ribs with each inhalation as the air is
drawn more into that side of the chest and it is exercised fully.

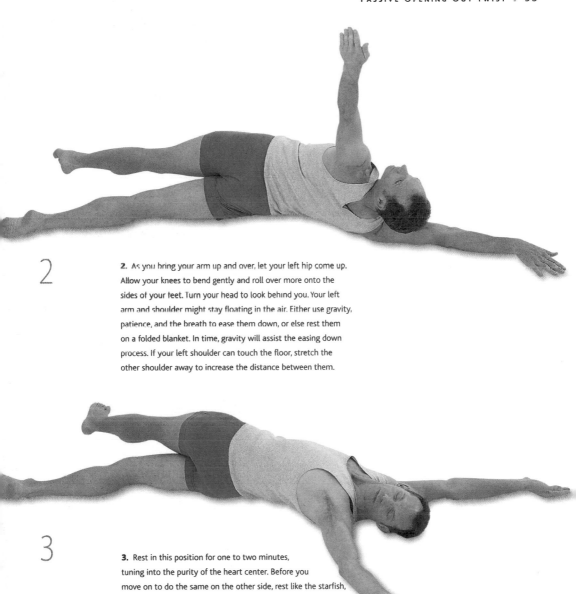

2

2. As you bring your arm up and over, let your left hip come up. Allow your knees to bend gently and roll over more onto the sides of your feet. Turn your head to look behind you. Your left arm and shoulder might stay floating in the air. Either use gravity, patience, and the breath to ease them down, or else rest them on a folded blanket. In time, gravity will assist the easing down process. If your left shoulder can touch the floor, stretch the other shoulder away to increase the distance between them.

3

3. Rest in this position for one to two minutes, tuning into the purity of the heart center. Before you move on to do the same on the other side, rest like the starfish, or in Makrasana (see page 125) to observe what has been mobilized on the physical, mental, and/or emotional levels.

MARICHYASANA III SAGE TWIST III

30

This twist develops shoulder flexibility, tones the abdominal organs, and stimulates sluggish intestinal function. This pose is named after Marichi, who, like Bharadvaja, was a man of great wisdom.

1. Sit in Dandasana (*see* page 54). Bend the left knee so that your heel comes close to your buttock. Before planting the seed of "twisting" in the mind, allow yourself to grow taller. Lean back on your left hand and reach your right hand up to the sky. Take as many breaths as necessary to "grow" both sides of the torso.

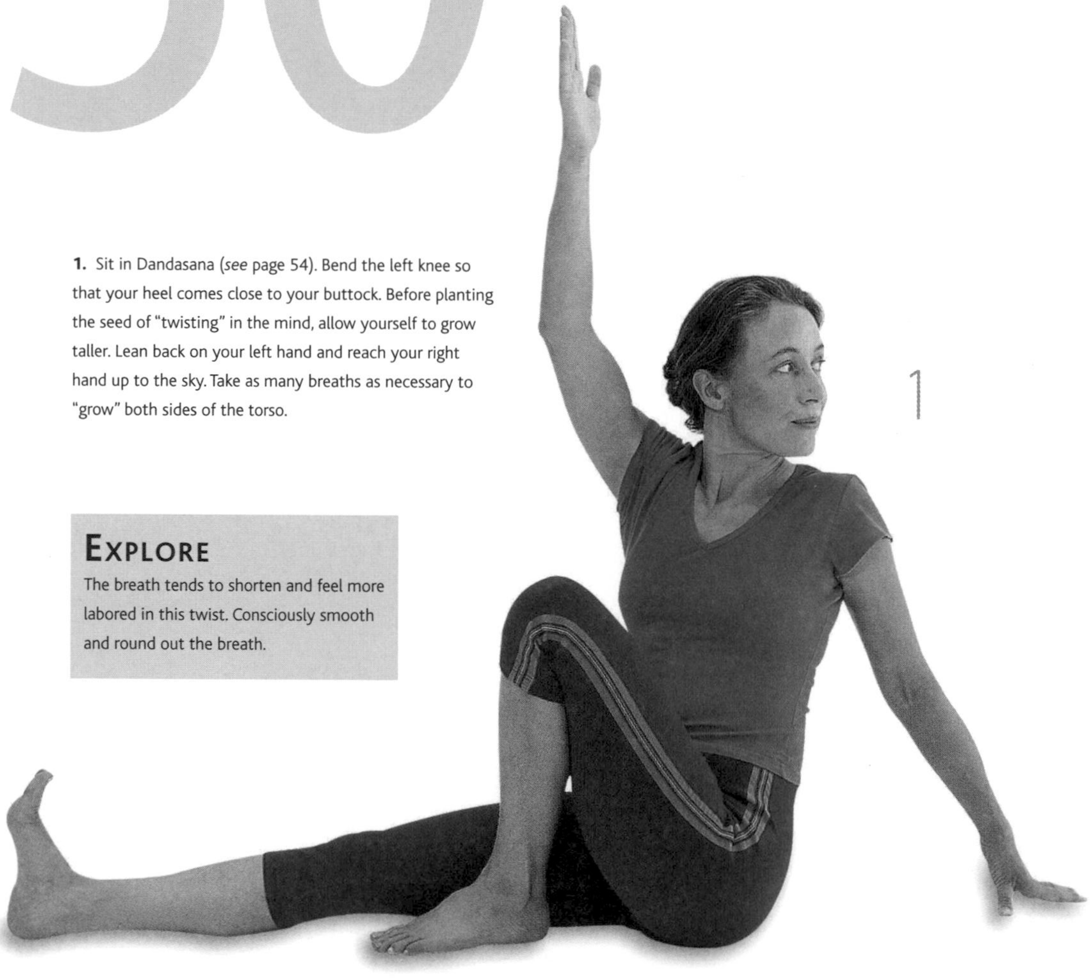

EXPLORE

The breath tends to shorten and feel more labored in this twist. Consciously smooth and round out the breath.

1

2. This next part is crucial. You need to lean forward and wedge your right elbow to the left outer knee without losing the length you have just gained. Do this movement consciously, over one or more exhalations, taking care not to shorten the left side of the torso. Twist in sections from the base up. Twist on the exhale until you reach the chest, and then twist on the inhale. Feel yourself twisting from the inside out; from the inner organs to the outer casing of your body. Hold for five to ten breaths, then untwist, recenter, and repeat on the other side.

2

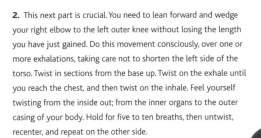

3. For the full posture, straighten your left arm forward. Reach well forward as if you were taking your armpit beyond the left outer knee. From the shoulder, rotate the whole arm so that the thumb turns down, and wrap your arm around the left knee. Clasp the right wrist behind your back, or work your hands toward each other using a soft belt. As you breathe deeply in this pose, the pressure of your thigh against your abdomen gives the organs a healthy massage.

3

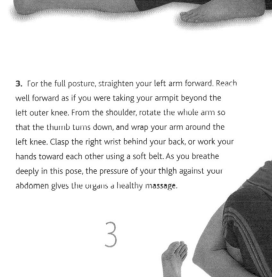

BALANCES

Our lives feel better when they are well balanced. We are healthiest when we find the appropriate balance in the food we eat. We feel best when we find the right levels of activity and sleep. Intellectual balance means we are able to see both sides of the coin, and be less judgmental.

Emotionally, we seek to lessen extremes of emotions, decrease mood swings, and be more even tempered. Spiritual balance lets us keep higher ideals in mind as our actions create our lives, yet still allows us to keep our feet on the ground. A spiritual belief balances and gives meaning to our physical existence. Being out of balance is a huge source of stress and tends to create problems. Your yoga practice is a metaphor for your life. Finding your balance in a pose is practice at finding your balance in your life. Yoga, as a reharmonizer, helps you move closer to your own perfect balance.

Balance poses convey self-sufficiency. Standing on your own two feet does more than just develop the small muscles of the ankles. Balancing poses allow us to explore our connection with our base. In India, the lotus flower is a powerful symbol. The white flower is a symbol of purity. It floats on top of its stem, a long taproot that is anchored in deep, dark waters. Like the lotus flower, we sink our roots into the earth, and soar skyward. Balance poses allow you to connect to your roots and explore whether they feel strong, independent, and able to support your growth.

Some poses look simple but actually present a real challenge. All balance poses require that the mind and body work together. The focused mind collaborates with the grounded body. Aside from developing concentration and stamina, the poses develop patience. Don't be in a hurry. Decide for how many breaths you will stay in the pose, then stay. If you come out early, keep a quiet mind and bring yourself back into it again.

Arm balances develop endurance. They work the shoulder girdle, which helps balance out office-bound people. By building strength in the upper body, they redistribute tension in a healthy way, which helps decrease neck tension. Developing the arms enables us to reach out in life, either to take what we need or to give what we can.

Balance poses teach us about relaxing in all the other postures. Try balancing when holding your body tight. It will feel very different from when you proceed in a soft, easy manner that brings a lightness into your pose. Use the skeleton rather than tensed muscles to support you. As your mind stays calm and centered and develops the ability to lead the body, your coordination will grow. Developing physical poise will foster mental harmony.

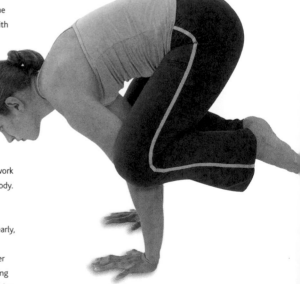

Above and opposite: *Being out of balance creates stress. Yoga practice helps you move closer to a balanced way of living.*

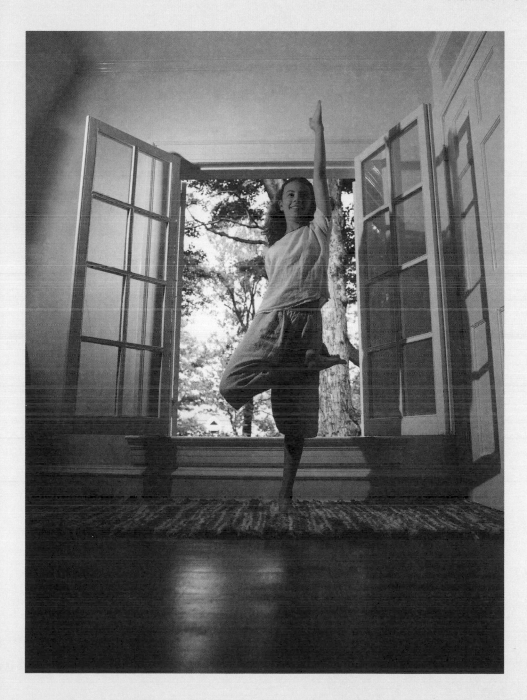

UTTHITA HASTA PADANGUSTHASANA

HAND TO FOOT POSE

When a balance pose is a challenge to flexibility, it is amazing how we are forced to focus to stay up. This is good practice.

1. Stand in Tadasana (*see* page 38) and ground yourself through your heels. Quiet the mind so that you can fully focus on what you are doing right here and now: this balance. Gaze at a fixed point at eye level. Bend the right knee slightly and pause tolet your left leg better connect with the earth. Lift up your right leg and hold the knee with your right hand. With your left hand to your hip, lift the sternum so that your posture stays erect. Lengthen the right-side waist by moving the right hip down, level with the left. Pressing the knee closer to the torso, hold for seven even breaths.

2. Now open the leg out to the right. Roving eyes will distract you by taking your awareness elsewhere. Turn your head to gaze left and keep your eyes steady. If you are holding your knee, lift it toward your armpit. If you are holding your toe (*see* alternative opposite), lift it as high as you can. Keep the supporting leg straight. Breathe here for seven rounds. Then, still balancing, bring the leg back to the front. Release the leg and straighten it in midair. Lower the leg slowly and practice the other side.

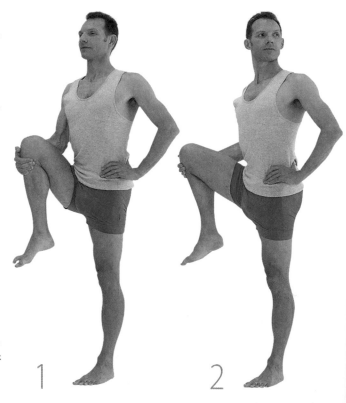

1

2

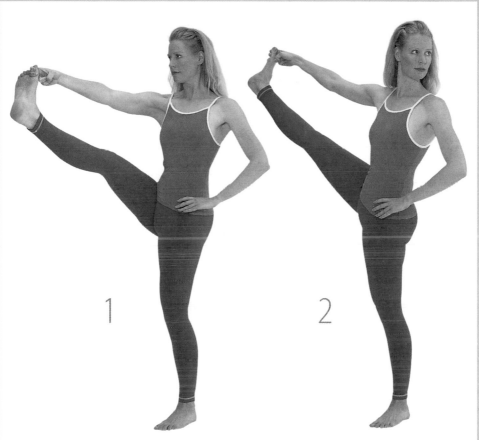

1

2

ALTERNATIVE

If your hamstrings are flexible, loop your big toe with the thumb and finger and straighten
the leg out in front (1). Now keep both sides of the torso an even length by rolling the
outer right hip down with an external rotation of the thigh bone (2).

CAUTION

During pregnancy, practice standing
balances near a wall so there is no risk
of falling.

EXPLORE

To build hamstring flexibility, stand in front of a table and
place your heel on it. Level the hips by lowering the raised
leg side.

GARUDASANA EAGLE POSE

This pose develops concentration and coordination and is wonderful for tight shoulders.

EXPLORE

Feel free to practice the upper and lower body movements independently, before uniting them in Garudasana.

1. From Tadasana (*see* page 38), become aware of the skin on the soles of the feet widening out against the floor. Move your attention to the pressure of the right foot against the floor. Quietly let the skin of the foot melt down into it. Bend the left knee and lift up the right leg.

2. Use momentum to wrap the right leg around the left leg. If you have difficulty with this, bend the supporting leg more. If possible, keep the top knee facing forward, not turned outward. To wrap the arms, hug yourself with your left arm on top of the right. Keeping the cross at the elbows, bring the backs of the hands toward each other, then cross wrist and forearm to bring the palms together.

3. Lift the elbows up so they rise off the chest and free breath is not impeded. To stretch into the shoulders more, ease your forearms forward so your thumbs move away from your nose. Let your eagle fold forward, as if looking down on the world from a great height. When you breathe deeply, you will feel the skin between the shoulder blades stretch on each inhalation. Hold the pose for ten breaths, before unwrapping, regrounding, and repeating on the opposite side.

1

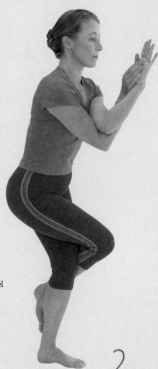

2

VIRABHADRASANA III WARRIOR III

Let your warrior-like
determination give you
a mental surge to charge
the body with energy.

1. Assume the pose for Virabhadrasana I with your right foot forward (*see* page 40).

2. Inhale deeply and, on the exhalation, fold your torso over your front leg, lowering your ribs towards your thigh. On a strong inhalation, straighten the right leg and lift the back leg up to parallel with the floor. Gaze straight ahead. Keeping your right leg straight, lower your left hip down so it is even with the right. Turn your left toes from the side down towards the floor and extend back through the heel. (You can even place your hands on the back of a chair to practice the alignment.) Visualize a line of energy running along the body. From the back of the waist it extends forward, reaching out towards the fingertips. From your center, it extends backwards through the back heel, so everything from heel to fingertips unkinks and elongates. Hold for five breaths before coming gracefully back to Virabhadrasana I.

EXPLORE

Before coming into a pose, close your eyes and visualize yourself clearly in a strong, stable, steady pose.

34

BHUJAPIDASANA

ARM PRESSURE BALANCE

Despite appearances, this pose doesn't require more upper-body strength than you already have. Technique is all-important. With attention to proper positioning and a positive mental attitude, you will be well on your way to balancing.

EXPLORE

Should your wrists need strengthening, practice Adho Mukha Svanasana (see page 106). To counterstretch the arms after Bhujapidasana, Bakasana or Adho Mukha Svanasana, kneel and place the backs of the hands on the floor, fingers facing towards your knees. Move the hips back about 5 cm (2 in). Feel the welcome release along the wrists and forearms as you lean back.

1. Stand with the feet hip-width apart. As you fold forward, bend the knees but keep your hips high in the air. Take the right arm through the legs and around the right leg. A common error is not to take the whole arm – up to the shoulder – through the legs. It is important that the back of the thigh contacts as high up the upper arm as possible so use your other hand to stabilize you if necessary. Place the right palm flat on the floor just next to the right foot, with fingers facing forward. Now take the left arm through to bring that palm flat to the floor. You'll need to keep the hips high so you don't squash your upper arm and get stuck halfway in, unable to proceed.

2. Bending your elbows well, lean forward. Inch your feet together and forward. Lift up through the abdominal region and raise your head to gaze forward. Shift your weight to transfer more weight to the palms as you lift your feet up in the air to cross the ankles. Straighten the arms and hold for five to ten breaths. After resting, repeat with the feet crossed the opposite way.

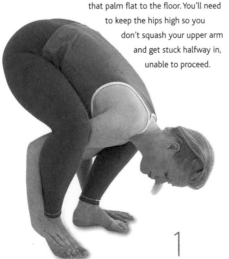

1

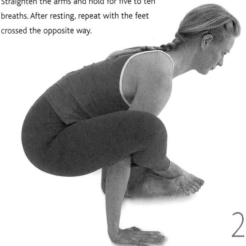

2

35 BAKASANA CRANE POSE

This pose, resembling a bird, strengthens the upper body and abdomen.

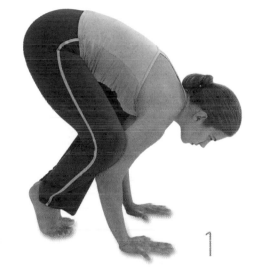

1. Squat with your feet together. Place your hands on the floor as wide as your shoulders, middle fingers facing forward. Bend your knees to rest them high up the upper arms, wrapping your inner knees around the upper arms. Bring the feet together and come onto your tiptoes.

2. Lean forward to allow the transfer of weight from toes to palms. Gaze forward along the floor. Lift the abdominal muscles and use yogic energy locks to give your body lift and lightness. One at a time, or together, raise the feet toward the buttocks. Keep your abdominal muscles contracted to help draw the legs into the body. Straighten your arms. Take five breaths before coming down with control.

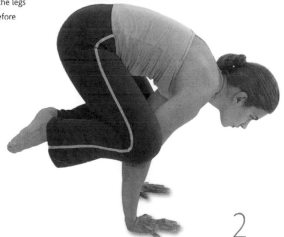

EXPLORE

As you commit to a pose, you agree to go on a journey and appreciate what it has to offer you. When practicing balancing poses, decide first for how many breaths you will stay and keep to it.

INVERSIONS

Holding a position with a whole new relationship to gravity demands a certain steadiness of posture and mind. Inversions develop confidence and help quiet the brain in times of stress.

Inversions are key poses for regaining hormonal balance, as better blood circulation tones the endocrine glands. In particular, Headstand tones the pituitary and pineal glands in the brain, both of which have wide-ranging effects in the body. Shoulderstand and Plough Pose bring blood to the thyroid and parathyroid glands by the throat.

The lymphatic system, involved in immune support and clearing toxins from the tissues, reaps the benefits from antigravity positions. The lymphatic vessels don't have any valves or muscles to help pump their fluid through. The passive flow instead relies on changes in position and massaging movements from the muscles surrounding them. Going upside down helps

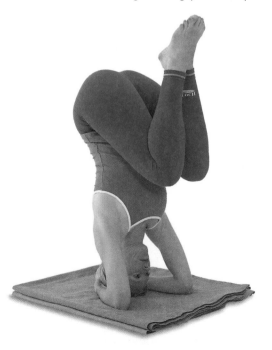

drain toxins from the extremities down toward their destination: the lymph nodes. The lymphatic fluid drains in the direction of the heart and, by assisting this process, inverted poses relieve strain or swelling in the legs and clear the path for improved blood circulation.

Inversions are even considered aerobic, as the heart must pump harder to pump out the more rapidly filling ventricles. The functioning of the organs is stimulated by the change in position and circulation, and intestinal laziness is lessened by the alteration in internal pressure.

When you feel stuck, or in need of inspiration, it helps to see the world from another angle. Releasing the pressure of our normal reality—gravity—can lighten the mind, too. An upside-down position is an opportunity to consider things from a different point of view. Apart from being mentally revitalizing and rejuvenating, inversions have the same physical action. By cleansing and nourishing the tissues, many people swear by their effects at maintaining youthfulness. As a sort of holistic beauty treatment, they might be the closest you can get to turning back the clock.

If you suffer high blood pressure, a neck problem, eye, ear, or sinus problems, heart problems, hiatus hernia, or dizzy spells, seek advice from a medical practitioner or experienced yoga teacher before beginning inversions. During pregnancy, work with an experienced teacher. Inversions are not advisable during menstruation, as they tend to slow down the flow of blood. Don't practice inverted poses if you have a headache at the time. As inversions are considered calming to the mind and cooling to the system, they are generally used toward the end of your asana practice, and when your body has been warmed by the other poses.

Above and opposite: Inverted poses clear the head and help concentration. The brain receives an increased blood supply, combating tiredness and lethargy.

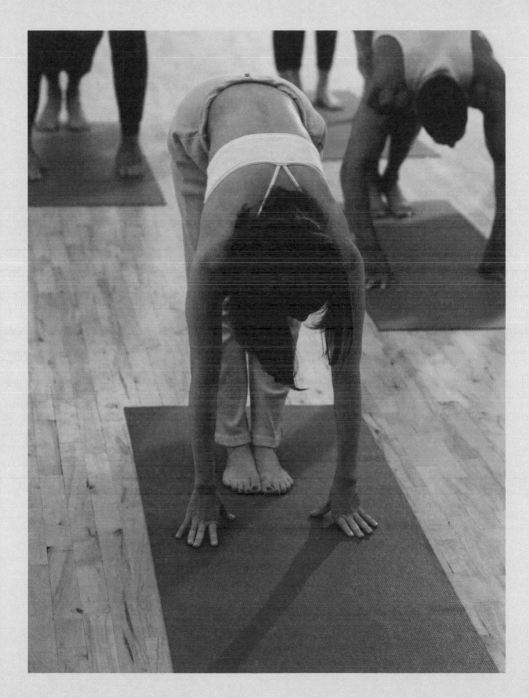

ADHO MUKHA SVANASANA

DOWNWARD-FACING DOG

This is an excellent pose for stretching and strengthening the whole body. This forward-folding mild inversion is useful to link standing poses. Although it may not feel very restful at first, it can become so when you develop strength and flexibility.

If, instead of being relatively straight, your back rounds in the full Downward-Facing Dog, practice Puppy Dog. As a gentler way to open the shoulders, you can hold and breathe in this pose longer. If wrist problems prevent you doing the full pose at this time, begin with this easier version.

1

1. Begin on all fours with your hands placed about 6 in (15 cm) in front of the shoulders. Check that the middle finger is pointing straight ahead, and spread the fingers wide.

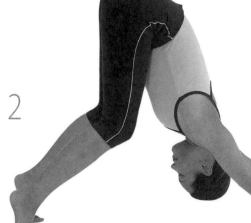

2

2. Have your knees and feet body-width apart. Tuck the toes under and lift up to an inverted "V" position. On tiptoes, bend both knees deeply, so your ribs come toward the thighs, or even touch. You will feel an increase in the stretch through the shoulders and an opening in the chest. At the same time, lift the sitting bones as the buttocks stay high and tilt the pelvis forward. The inward curve in the lower back will deepen as your navel moves closer to your thighs. (This pose is also a forward bend, so refresh your body's memory about folding from the hips: *see* page 39.) You will feel the muscles along the spine working strongly and get a lifting sense of elongation along the spine.

3. Keeping the hips at the same height, slowly straighten the legs. If the hips stay at, or nearly at, the same height, everything in between will need to lengthen. Practice this several times, with full awareness, so you don't lose the feeling of height or the inward curve in the lower back. To complete, swivel your feet so the outside edges of your feet are parallel—the inner heels will be farther away from each

other than the big toes. Stretch your heels toward the ground (until you develop a lot of flexibility along the backs of the legs, they will remain in the air). Distribute the pressure equally through the whole palm and fingers. Widen the space between the earlobes and upper arms by turning the outer edges of the armpits in toward each other. Hold for ten to 15 breaths. Rest in Child Pose (see page 23) afterward. Soften the arms from the shoulders all the way to the wrists. To release the wrists, follow the instructions on page 102.

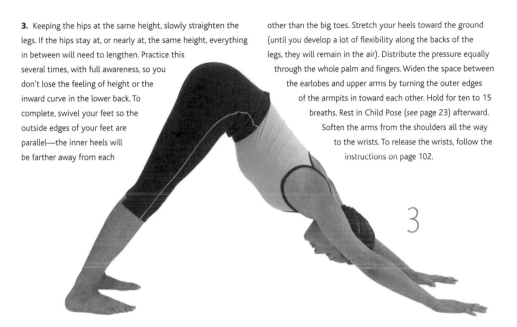

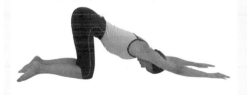

ALTERNATIVE Puppy Dog

This gentler version of Downward-Facing Dog gives the shoulders a good stretch. Kneel on the floor. Place your hands far forward and lower your forehead to the floor. Have your knees under your hips so your buttocks are high in the air, not near the heels. From the back of the waist, extend back strongly through the tailbone. At the same time direct your energy from the waist forward through the arms.

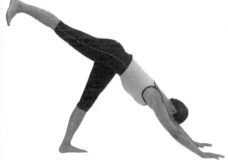

ALTERNATIVE Raised-Leg Variation

To make this pose into a stronger inversion, start with your feet together. Turn the right toes out and lift the right leg high up in the air. Keep both shoulders level. Let your right hip rise and extend back through both heels. After five to ten breaths, lower the leg and stretch through both legs (or rest in Child Pose— see page 23) before practicing the other side.

SIRSASANA HEADSTAND

37

Your head weighs about 9 lb (4 kg), your body considerably more. Your neck can hold the weight of your head only when you are properly prepared. It is essential to understand the lifting through the shoulders and pay due attention to alignment. This is not a beginner's pose and I strongly recommend you ask an experienced teacher to observe your alignment. If Headstand is not yet for you, the Hare Pose (*see* page 111) is a possible alternative.

Headstand is a yogic icon, often the first pose people think of when they first hear of yoga. Ironically, you must get your head out of the way in Headstand. If you want to do this classic pose just because your ego wants to do "real yoga," it doesn't necessarily mean your body is ready to follow. Practice Headstand well into your practice when your body is warm. Before going up, visualize yourself in the posture. Form a clear picture of yourself in a steady, stable pose.

1. Always practice Headstand on a cushioned surface like a folded blanket. Place your blanket in front of a wall, or in the corner of two walls. Kneel in front of your blanket. To measure out the correct elbow-width, place your forearms on the blanket and cup each elbow in the opposite hand. Your elbows should be not wider than your shoulders. Then form your triangle of support by interlacing your fingers. Your knuckles should be 2 in (5 cm) from the wall.

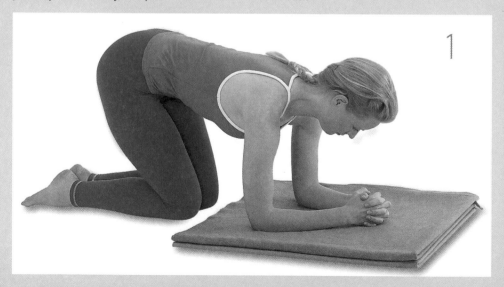

1

2. When performing a safe Headstand, it is crucial to lift well from elbows to shoulders. Tuck your toes under and straighten your knees so that you are in an inverted "V" shape. Practice your lift by pressing down through the elbows and moving the shoulders up toward the hips. This movement should increase the distance between the shoulders and earlobes as well as lifting the head away from the floor. If you find you can't lift your head away from the floor, you are not ready for Headstand yet. You need to develop your shoulder flexibility and/or strength before attempting to go up into Headstand. For shoulder flexibility, practice the shoulder exercises on page 73, as well as Gomukhasana (*see* page 66), and Garudasana (*see* page 100). To develop arm strength, practice Downward-Facing Dog (*see* page 106).

3. Take your knees back to the floor and position your head on the floor to be cupped by your interlaced fingers. For the correct alignment in the neck, it is the crown of the head that should be in contact with the floor. Once again raise the knees off the floor and practice moderating the pressure on the head. Ground down through the elbows, distribute weight into the edges of the hands against the floor, lift the shoulders up toward the hips. If you are not able to minimize the pressure on the crown of the head with these actions, then don't move on to the next step. Develop this skill with more preparatory work before you come up into Headstand.

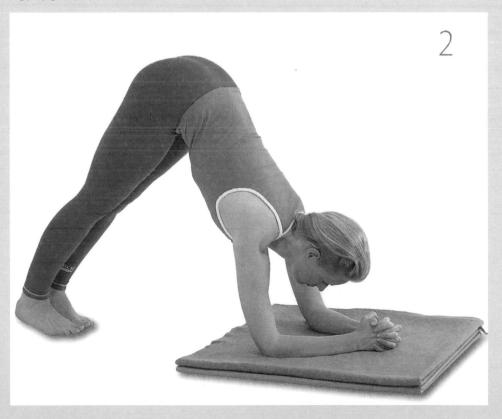

2

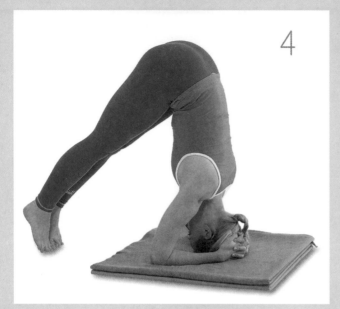

4

4. If you have passed these checks, then walk your feet in as much as possible. There will come a point where the feet naturally want to lift. Lift them with knees bent so your heels come near your buttocks. Don't raise the legs all the way up straight away. Follow these steps to help your alignment stay true. Lift up from your elbows through your shoulders to your hips once more.

5. If you are not using a wall and feel balanced, keep your knees bent and raise the thighs so the knees point upward. Your heels will still be near your buttocks. Then straighten your legs up. If you are by a wall, straighten your legs and lift upward through the balls of the feet.

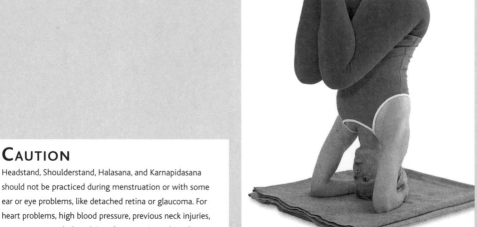

5

CAUTION

Headstand, Shoulderstand, Halasana, and Karnapidasana should not be practiced during menstruation or with some ear or eye problems, like detached retina or glaucoma. For heart problems, high blood pressure, previous neck injuries, or pregnancy, seek the advice of an experienced teacher.

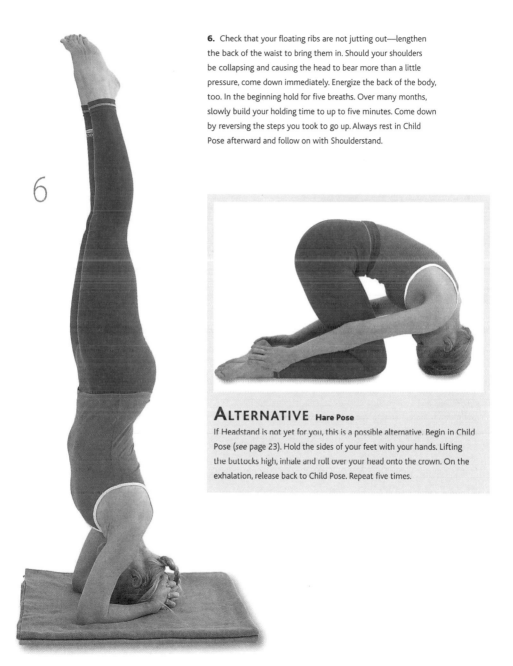

6. Check that your floating ribs are not jutting out—lengthen the back of the waist to bring them in. Should your shoulders be collapsing and causing the head to bear more than a little pressure, come down immediately. Energize the back of the body, too. In the beginning hold for five breaths. Over many months, slowly build your holding time to up to five minutes. Come down by reversing the steps you took to go up. Always rest in Child Pose afterward and follow on with Shoulderstand.

ALTERNATIVE Hare Pose

If Headstand is not yet for you, this is a possible alternative. Begin in Child Pose (see page 23). Hold the sides of your feet with your hands. Lifting the buttocks high, inhale and roll over your head onto the crown. On the exhalation, release back to Child Pose. Repeat five times.

SARVANGASANA SHOULDERSTAND

This hormonal balancing and deeply calming pose is well worth practicing daily.

1. To keep your neck relaxed in this pose, fold two or three blankets to the size that will support your base. Place the folded edges neatly, one on top of the other. Lie over them with your head on the lower level and the tops of your shoulders on your blankets, 2 in (5 cm) from the edge.

2. With control, bring your legs and hips in the air and then support your back. If your stomach muscles are not yet strong enough to bring you up, or if you can't yet come up in a well-controlled way that feels safe, use the wall method. Once you are up, bend your knees toward your head. Take several breaths to settle your shoulders into the pose. Let yourself come more onto the tips of the well-grounded shoulders and walk the hands down your back. Finally, stretch your legs up into the air. In the beginning, your legs may be angled to be quite bent overhead, not straight up in the air. Bring your elbows closer together. You may get a better grip holding your palms against the skin on your back rather than your clothes. In time, work on lessening the crease where the thighs join the torso. Visualize a line of energy from the inner thigh to the inner heel.

1

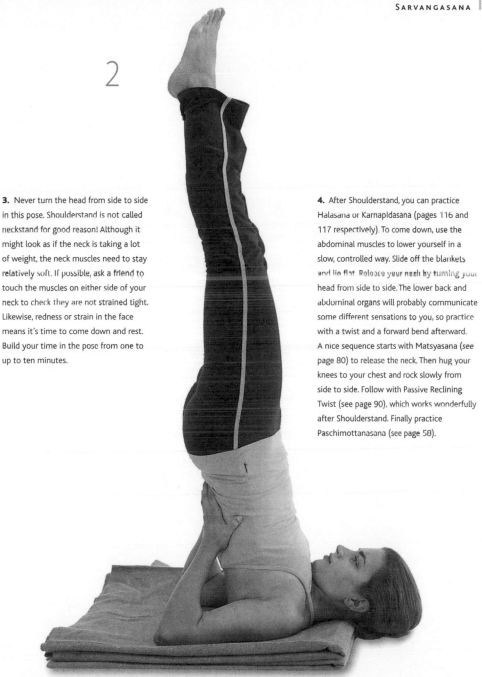

2

3. Never turn the head from side to side in this pose. Shoulderstand is not called neckstand for good reason! Although it might look as if the neck is taking a lot of weight, the neck muscles need to stay relatively soft. If possible, ask a friend to touch the muscles on either side of your neck to check they are not strained tight. Likewise, redness or strain in the face means it's time to come down and rest. Build your time in the pose from one to up to ten minutes.

4. After Shoulderstand, you can practice Halasana or Karnapidasana (pages 116 and 117 respectively). To come down, use the abdominal muscles to lower yourself in a slow, controlled way. Slide off the blankets and lie flat. Release your neck by turning your head from side to side. The lower back and abdominal organs will probably communicate some different sensations to you, so practice with a twist and a forward bend afterward. A nice sequence starts with Matsyasana (see page 80) to release the neck. Then hug your knees to your chest and rock slowly from side to side. Follow with Passive Reclining Twist (see page 90), which works wonderfully after Shoulderstand. Finally practice Paschimottanasana (see page 58).

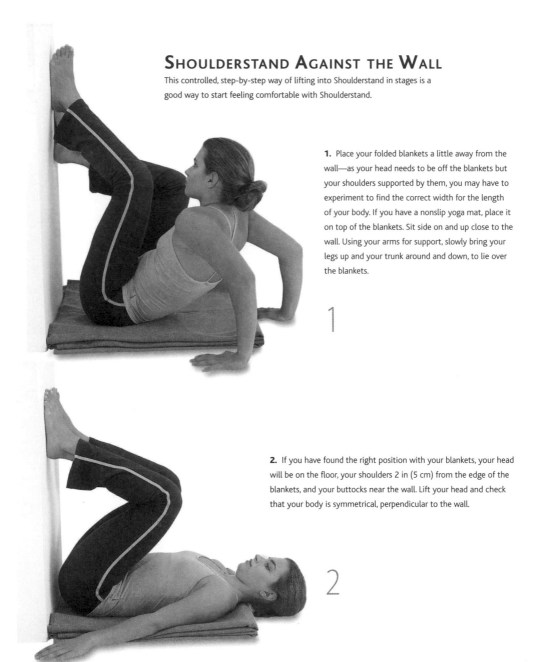

SHOULDERSTAND AGAINST THE WALL

This controlled, step-by-step way of lifting into Shoulderstand in stages is a good way to start feeling comfortable with Shoulderstand.

1. Place your folded blankets a little away from the wall—as your head needs to be off the blankets but your shoulders supported by them, you may have to experiment to find the correct width for the length of your body. If you have a nonslip yoga mat, place it on top of the blankets. Sit side on and up close to the wall. Using your arms for support, slowly bring your legs up and your trunk around and down, to lie over the blankets.

1

2. If you have found the right position with your blankets, your head will be on the floor, your shoulders 2 in (5 cm) from the edge of the blankets, and your buttocks near the wall. Lift your head and check that your body is symmetrical, perpendicular to the wall.

2

3. Now you are ready to come up! With knees bent, press your feet into the wall and lift your hips. Hold your back and straighten yourself up by moving your hips more in line over your shoulders. If you like, you can straighten each leg in turn, bringing one foot up the wall. Once you have both legs straight against the wall, take one leg, then the other, overhead and away from the wall. Come down by reversing the steps you took to go up.

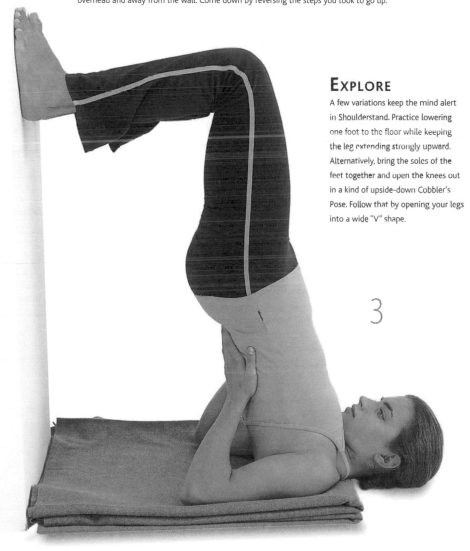

EXPLORE

A few variations keep the mind alert in Shoulderstand. Practice lowering one foot to the floor while keeping the leg extending strongly upward. Alternatively, bring the soles of the feet together and open the knees out in a kind of upside-down Cobbler's Pose. Follow that by opening your legs into a wide "V" shape.

3

HALASANA PLOUGH POSE

39

If you are comfortable in Shoulderstand, follow on with this soothing pose. It has similar effects and contraindications to Shoulderstand.

1. From Shoulderstand lower your legs overhead. You need to be careful not to overstretch the neck as you bring your toes to touch the floor. If you are not able to bring your toes to the floor, then rest them on a higher surface, such as a chair placed a couple of feet behind the head. (If your toes are not supported, then continue to support your back with your hands.)

2. Once your toes are resting on a surface, stretch your arms along the floor. This will help you roll more onto the tips of your shoulders and deeper into this upside-down forward bend. Interlace your fingers and deepen the pose by stretching your arms and legs in opposite directions. Build up to holding this pose for five minutes. Make Plough Pose more restful by supporting the thighs with a chair if you wish.

3. Roll out of the pose with control, using your abdominal muscles to lower both legs until you are lying flat. See Shoulderstand for complementary asanas to follow on with.

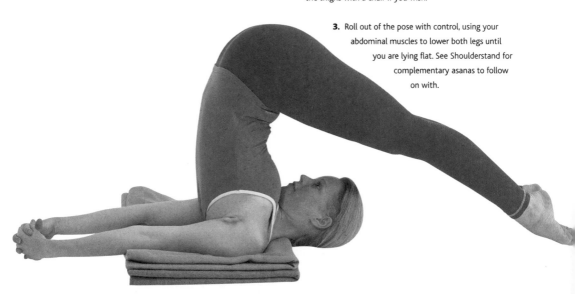

KARNAPIDASANA KNEE TO EAR POSE

40

Withdraw into a fetal position after practicing
Shoulderstand and Plough Pose.

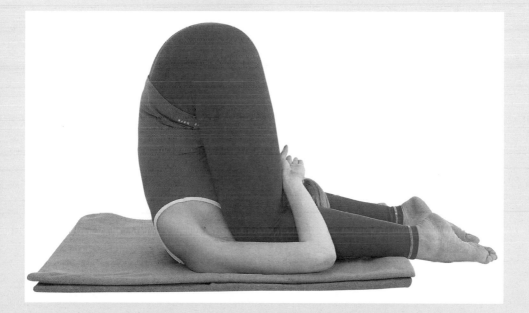

If you feel comfortable in Halasana, practice this deep forward stretch by cushioning yourself with a couple of folded blankets and bending your knees beside your head. If your knees and the tops of the feet don't come to the floor, place your legs on raised supports or tuck your toes under if necessary.

To deepen the pose, straighten both arms along the floor and interlace your fingers. If your knees touch the floor, fold your arms over the backs of your knees. Hold this pose for ten to 20 breaths before coming back to Halasana.

SURYA NAMASKAR

SUN SALUTATION

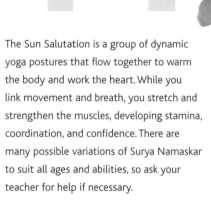

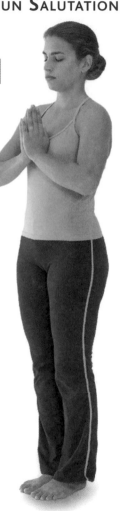

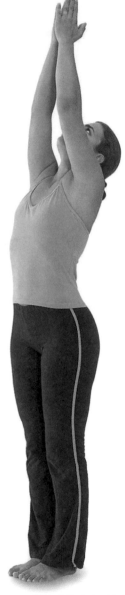

1

2

The Sun Salutation is a group of dynamic yoga postures that flow together to warm the body and work the heart. While you link movement and breath, you stretch and strengthen the muscles, developing stamina, coordination, and confidence. There are many possible variations of Surya Namaskar to suit all ages and abilities, so ask your teacher for help if necessary.

The sun is a symbol of the inner light that is in all of us. The bowing is an exercise of deep respect for this shining light, the folding and unfolding movements a tribute to creation. As you develop a graceful flow of one movement per breath, it becomes a moving meditation. Start your practice with three rounds and build to six, offering each one up like a prayer. Then sit quietly and listen as your body tells you what it would like to practice next.

1. Mountain Pose with palms together, ground through the feet and feel the connection with the earth through the soles of the feet.

2. Inhale your arms skyward. As the front of your torso lengthens, keep the back side of the torso long as well.

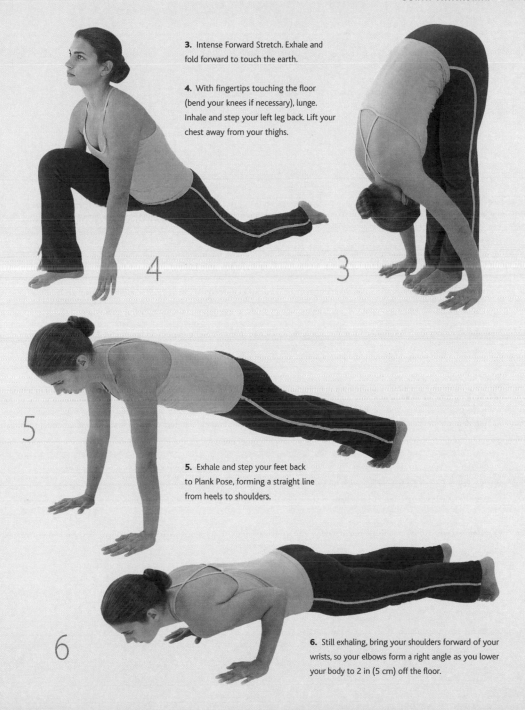

3. Intense Forward Stretch. Exhale and fold forward to touch the earth.

4. With fingertips touching the floor (bend your knees if necessary), lunge. Inhale and step your left leg back. Lift your chest away from your thighs.

5. Exhale and step your feet back to Plank Pose, forming a straight line from heels to shoulders.

6. Still exhaling, bring your shoulders forward of your wrists, so your elbows form a right angle as you lower your body to 2 in (5 cm) off the floor.

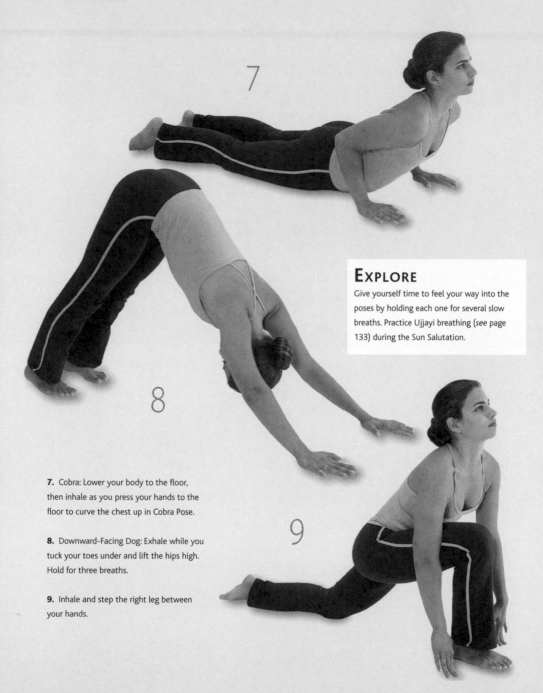

7

8

9

EXPLORE

Give yourself time to feel your way into the poses by holding each one for several slow breaths. Practice Ujjayi breathing (*see* page 133) during the Sun Salutation.

7. Cobra: Lower your body to the floor, then inhale as you press your hands to the floor to curve the chest up in Cobra Pose.

8. Downward-Facing Dog: Exhale while you tuck your toes under and lift the hips high. Hold for three breaths.

9. Inhale and step the right leg between your hands.

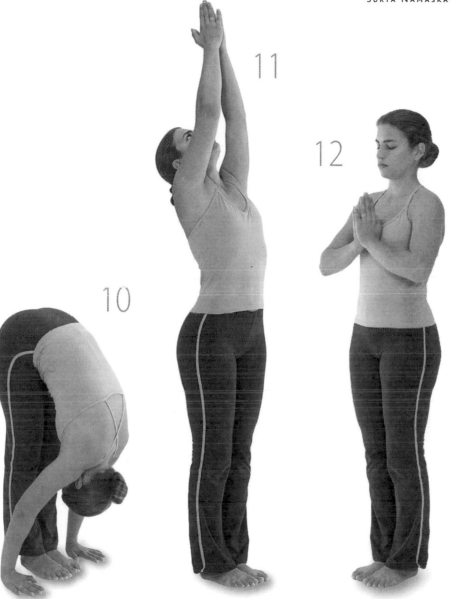

10. Intense Forward Stretch. Exhale as you step your left leg forward, then fold over your legs. If your legs are straight, press your hands more to the floor.

11. Switch on your thigh muscles and those of the lower abdomen as you inhale skyward. Lift everything from the hips up, except the shoulders.

12. Exhale and bring the arms down to Mountain Pose, ready to repeat on the left side.

RESTORATIVE YOGA

Restorative poses open the body, yet allow the nervous system to rest. Though you can still stretch deeply, the support helps you feel safe and comfortable yielding to the pose, and you can stay in it for longer. It enables you to recharge by expending minimal energy.

As such, these poses are wonderful should you need to build energy stores during a chronic illness, or to tap into your inner reserves and rejuvenate whenever you feel depleted.

Incorporate restorative poses into your regular practice routine, either by practicing them a few days each month (they are ideal during menstruation), or by bringing one or two poses into each more active practice session.

To find props around your house, think creatively and use sofa cushions, cushions, blankets, chairs, soft belts, and bathrobe ties. An eyebag gives the system a break from sensory overload.

SUPTA KONASANA

SUPPORTED ANGLE POSE

This restorative pose creates space in the pelvis, eases menstrual dysfunction for women, and supports the digestive system. It is worth folding a pile of blankets to luxuriate in complete comfort in this pose.

Use a bolster or fold up several blankets so they are longer than your torso. Sit at one end of your support and bring the soles of your feet together, heels toward your groin. Lie back over the bolster and have an extra cushion under your head so it is higher than the heart. Let your knees fall out to the sides and use pillows or folded blankets of equal heights to support your thighs. Find the right balance between opening the hips and staying comfortable—if the stretch becomes too intense it will be hard to rest. Cover your body for warmth if necessary. Lay your arms out to the sides, palms facing up. If your elbows don't naturally reach the floor, then fold towels or blankets to support the forearms. Close or cover your eyes and rest for five to ten minutes. When you come up, stretch forward in Child Pose, or a variation of it with your big toes together, knees apart and arms stretched forward.

FORWARD BEND WITH A CHAIR

The same principle can be used for many forward bends: Trianga Mukhaikapada Paschimottanasana, Janu Sirsasana, Ardha Baddha Padma Paschimottanasana, Paschimottanasana, and Baddha Konasana.

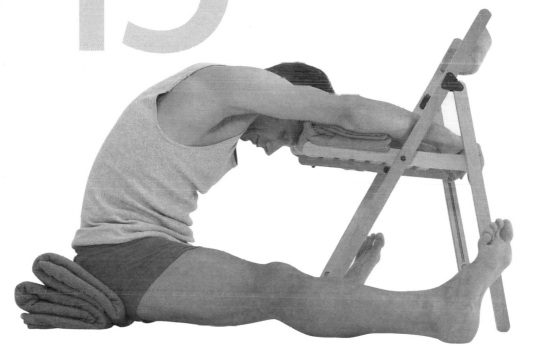

Sit on the edge of a folded blanket with your legs wide apart. Place a second blanket over the seat of a chair. Bring the chair far enough away so that when you fold forward, your forehead will rest on it. To keep the chest open, bring the arms up to hold the chair base or back—experiment to find the most comfortable position. If you feel too much stretch, use cushions to raise the level of your forehead. After some time in the pose, your body will release and you'll find you can slide the chair farther away

to deepen the stretch. If you are very flexible, then you can rest your forehead on just a bolster or cushions. The gentle pressure on the forehead rests the frontal lobe of the brain, helping to quieten the mind and soothe the soul. Next, in this resting variation of Upavista Konasana, you can do two twists, too. Turn your torso to face over one leg, position the chair over it and fold forward to rest the forehead. Hold each forward bend for one to two minutes.

VIPARITA KARANI

RESTORATIVE INVERSION

Viparita Karani is used to seal life energy in your body. Enjoy the benefits of an inversion without the effort of holding yourself in place. To relieve swelling in the legs after a hard day, or to ease the pain of varicose veins, practice for ten minutes every day. During menstruation, forgo the blankets and simply lie on the floor with the legs up the wall.

Take a bolster or fold several blankets and place them by a wall. To come into the position, sit on your prop and lie down on your side so your buttocks stay high and near the wall. Roll onto your back and take your legs up the wall. Check your position. Your abdomen needs to be parallel to the floor and your ribcage will curve downward. You may need to experiment a bit to get the right height and width in your blankets. If either is wrong, it will feel as if you might slide off and you won't be able to relax properly. When the position feels perfect, look along your body to check that your trunk is perpendicular to the wall. If you like, tie a soft belt around the mid-thighs so your legs don't have to work to hold their position. You can cover your eyes with an eyebag. Choose a comfortable arm position—either slightly away from your sides with your palms facing up, or with the arms overhead and elbows softly bent.

Rest and breathe.

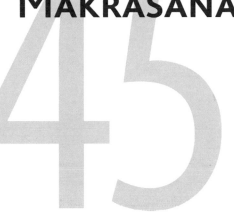

MAKRASANA CROCODILE POSE

This resting position has a gentle backbend, so it is useful for resting without breaking the flow in between stronger backbends. Experiment to find the angle of the upper arms that will give you the perfect feeling of the right amount of backbend and the right angle for the resting neck and head.

Lie face down with your feet wide apart and toes turned out. Cup each elbow in the opposite hand and slide the forearms away so they are a short distance in front of your shoulders. Lower your head to rest your forehead on your forearms. Each time you inhale, your abdomen will expand down into the earth. Become attuned to the soothing sensation of this massage. This position is also useful to feel the expansion and consolidation along the back of the torso with each breath.

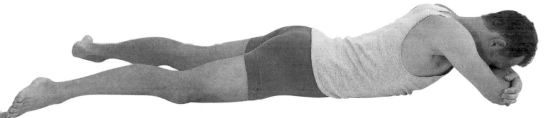

EXPLORE
A forward-bending restorative pose, which also creates a belly massage and permits the expansion of the back ribs, is Child Pose (see page 23).

NOTE
Savasana relaxation (see page 24), Discovering the Breath (see page 134), and letting yourself hang down in the Roll Downs (see page 34) are also restorative practices.

YOGA ON A CHAIR

These make great office exercises and they are also useful for the elderly or infirm. If you are at work, close the door and turn off your phone to give yourself the best chance for full mental relaxation.

BACKBEND

Different chairs will give you stretches of various intensities at different points along the spine, so experiment to find the best one for you. The chair back should be below or level with the lower part of your shoulder blades. If your chair is high-backed, sit on telephone books to raise your seat. Lift out of your hips and lean back over your chair. Let your head move back as you stretch your chin away. You can even sit with your back to the wall and find an angle to rest your head against the wall that provides complete relaxation.

Take the arms overhead and stretch them away like two rays of energy, to expand the backbend and make this stretch more invigorating. Take care that you do not slump—keep each vertebra actively lifting away from the one below it. Take five to ten chest-opening breaths.

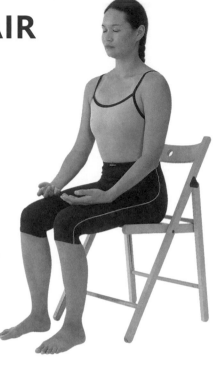

CENTERING

Sit comfortably on your chair. Have your feet well anchored to the ground. Bring the backs of your hands to your thighs. Sit with your back erect so you are not leaning against the backrest. Let your arms and shoulders relax and have your chin parallel to the floor. With each inhalation observe the expansion of the abdomen, ribs, and chest. The whole torso is alive with the gentle pulsation of the breath. Even the back of the body opens up, then softens inward rhythmically. Raise the inhalation from the back of the waist, upward. Each time you exhale feel the natural, passive release. As all heavy thoughts float away, the head will lighten so it feels as if it's floating happily on the top of your spine. The more you practice this, the quicker you will learn to recenter. Do it whenever you can throughout the day, letting tensions drift away as you return to your true, peaceful, inner self.

RELAXING FORWARD BEND

Sit on the chair with your feet body-width apart. If your feet don't touch
the floor easily, place a telephone book underfoot. Fold forward with
a flat back to lay your ribs on your thighs. Like a rag doll, your arms
hang out of their sockets, backs of the hands on the floor, fingers
softly curled. Your upper body grows heavier. Completely let
go of your head and shoulders so they release down toward
the floor. Any worries drop away. Now deepen the breath, so
the front of your torso expands into the thighs and the space
between them. Follow your exhalation for its entire length and
observe how it lengthens effortlessly. Stay like this for one to five
minutes before slowly coming up.

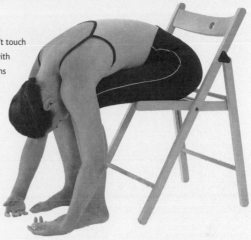

TWIST

Sit with your left hip to the back of the chair. Have your knees and feet hip-
width apart. Rest your feet on a support if they don't easily meet the ground.
Raise your arms straight up in the air. Let your torso rise out of your hips. Keep
this lift as you twist around to the left and hold the back of the chair. Work
from a steady base by keeping your hips and knees level. Twist progressively up
the spine. Stay for ten breaths before changing sides.

PALMING

Refresh with your own portable eyebag. Rub your hands together
so the friction builds heat. Rest your elbows on your desk and
rest your head in your hands, palms over your closed eyes. Lean
forward to apply a gentle pressure to your eyelids. Withdraw into
yourself and observe the wavelike rhythm of your breath.

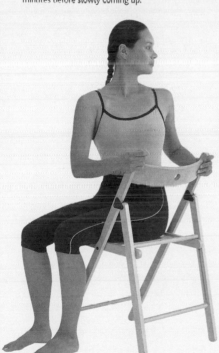

EXPLORE

Your body wants to move. It was made for it! Stretch anytime
using poles at bus stops, walls, or by grasping doorways to
hang forward to open the chest. While watching TV, sit on the
floor and notice that you naturally will want to stretch when
you change positions. Sit in front of the sofa and use it as a
back support for squatting or Cobbler's Pose (see page 62).

SHOULDER STRETCHES

The arm positions of Gomukhasana (see page 66), and
Garudasana (see page 100) can easily be practiced in a
chair and are great for those working in offices.

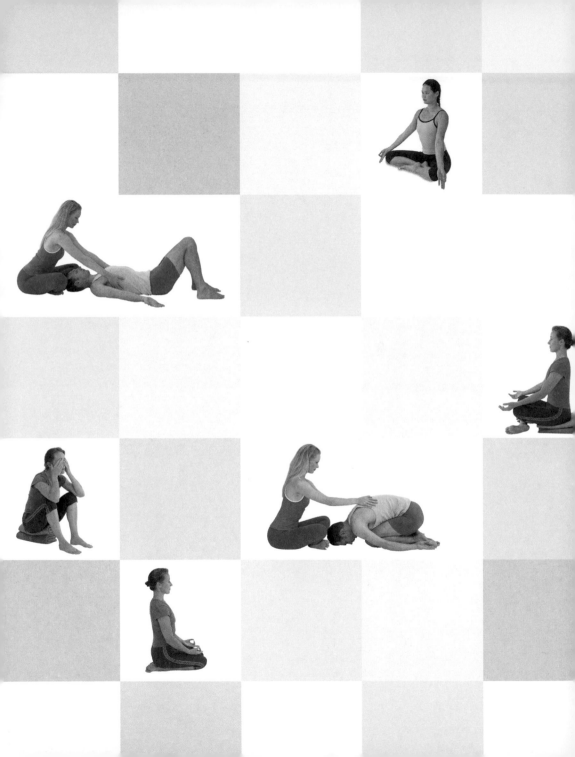

PRANAYAMA

PRANAYAMA

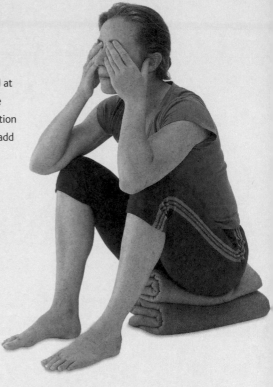

Have you ever watched children playing, and marveled at their endless energy? Have you ever felt that you were more tired than you should have been—as if the equation of energy expenditure versus remaining energy didn't add up?

People usually nominate food as the provider of our energy but we forget about a couple other important sources. Ideas, for one, supply us with boundless energy. You may have experienced being so taken with an idea that you were able to work late into the night without feeling fatigued. A third energy source, recognized by yogis for millennia, is the breath.

Breath, life, and energy are rooted together, and yogis have a single word for all three—"prana." Yogis consider death to occur when prana, the vital force, leaves the body. Conversely, when pranic levels are high, the body will be completely charged with energy. Pranayama may be translated either as restraint or control of the breath, or as pranic capacity. Pranayama exercises use breathing techniques to increase vitality and mental focus, and to expand consciousness.

Now become aware of your breath. Maintain this awareness until you have finished reading this introduction.

We don't have to think to breathe; it is instinctive and happens automatically. The breath is usually under the control of the medulla oblongata in the relatively primitive brain stem. During pranayama breathing, it shifts from being an involuntary and automatic process toward being more of a voluntary one, and it seems this activates the cerebral cortex, a more evolved part of the brain. Pranayama, by bringing a voluntary element to this involuntary process, has profound physiological, psychological, and spiritual effects.

Most simply, a breath is an intake of oxygen that gets distributed to our cells. The efficient, natural breath ensures that every cell in your body receives the energy it needs to do its job: digest, grow, heal, detoxify. Logically, a healthy body will be composed of well-nourished cells. Deep, conscious breathing, which fully expands the lungs, has an enormously positive impact on health and enhances all cellular processes. When we breathe better, we feel better.

When you touch a baby's belly, or a kitten's or puppy's, you can feel the whole torso moving completely freely. The chest and belly open and blossom with each breath. There is a delightful inner pulsation from expansion to consolidation, a sense of real freedom. However, as we move through life, we inevitably sustain some blows. Particularly as children, we have a limited capacity to understand. In response to the impacts of life, we form shielding patterns in our bodies. At some points, in some areas, our breath ceases to be the joyfully free flow it once was, and deviates into a new protective pattern. As adults we still breathe automatically and unconsciously, but due to our reactions to life, few of us breathe optimally. Those energetic children we were watching most likely still have relatively free breathing, responsive to the natural cues of the body.

Everything we do is affected by our breathing. The breath and the mind are intrinsically related; they are two expressions of the same entity. Think of the last time you felt angry or fearful: your breath became fast, shallow, and irregular. Compare this to when you were dozing in a comfortable chair. Probably your breath was deeper and slower. Just as your mind affects the breath, your breath affects the mind. Yogis have long recognized that when the breath becomes calm, the mind will, too. The *Hatha Yoga Pradipika*, an ancient text, tells us: "Respiration being disturbed, the mind becomes disturbed. By restraining respiration (pranayama), the Yogi attains steadiness of the mind."

The breath is a bridge to our nervous system, and enhanced breathing can improve our mental and emotional states. Firstly, by simply observing our breathing, we gain a mental point of focus that can quiet the constant chatter of the mind. Secondly, it relaxes the mind to promote clear thinking, decrease emotional fluctuations, and provide a sense of well-being. It is a valuable tool for self-management. Thirdly, like meditation, pranayama draws the senses inward, deepens awareness, and expands consciousness.

Conscious breathing encourages conscious action and conscious living in a calmer way. For returning to the self, we have been given the miracle of the breath. A good breathing habit is a wonderful ally in life, a valuable tool for self-management when dealing with confrontations, fear, agitation, anger, and confusion. Conscious breathing is certainly a mental challenge. Did you remember to be aware of your breath even as you were sitting reading?

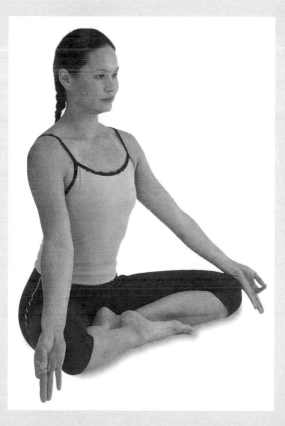

ABOUT PRACTICING

The exercises fall into two categories. During exercises in returning to the natural breath (*see* pages 30 and 134), you immerse yourself in your true breath and begin to disentangle it from any other superimposed breathing patterns. These exercises, where you don't add anything to your breath, are a great starting place. Release any pressure you may feel to breathe "correctly" or do it "the right way" and let your instincts take over. You can repeat them every day for weeks or months to get to know your breath, and return to them as often as you wish. The remaining exercises are pranayama, some of which lead on to more advanced practices involving alteration of the breath. If you wish to develop these further, the best way is to work alongside an experienced teacher.

Breath awareness and pranayama are fundamental. Ideally, they should be practiced daily. Just a few minutes will still be worthwhile. Use Savasana relaxation (*see* page 24) to separate pranayama and asana practice so that your energies settle.

CAUTION

Very deep inhalations should not be practiced if you have hypertension or heart problems. Extremely long exhalations are not advisable if you suffer from low blood pressure or depression.

HOW TO SIT

Our bodies are as individual as our personalities, so no single position reigns supreme for pranayama or meditation. There are really only two rules for sitting. The first is to sit erect so that your head, neck, and back are in line. The second is to be perfectly comfortable. Any physical discomfort will interfere with your concentration, alter your breath, and undo a little of your good work.

One of the things that makes pranayama special is that everyone can do it. If you can breathe, you can practice yoga! If you are ill or weak, lie down. You could use the breathing bed (*see* page 26) or, alternatively, let the torso soften down by lying flat and placing a bolster under your knees. Better still, keep yourself from drifting off to sleep by bending your knees, placing your feet on the floor a little wider than your hips, and letting the knees lean in together. If you find yourself getting sleepy, separate the knees.

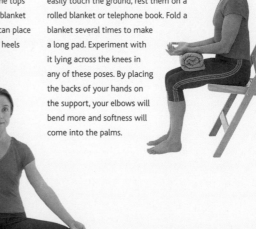

SUKHASANA
Comfortable Pose

Before practicing the cross-legged postures, use the leg cradling warm-up (*see* page 58) to unwind the leg at the hip socket. For Sukhasana, sit cross-legged and slide your feet apart so that each foot comes to rest underneath the opposite knee. It is difficult to sit upright with your shoulders over your hips if your knees are much higher than your hips. Use cushions or folded blankets to raise your seat if necessary.

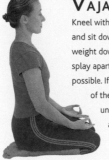

VAJARASANA Firm Pose

Kneel with your knees and ankles together and sit down on your heels. As you bring your weight down, your inner ankles will tend to splay apart. Keep them as close together as possible. If it causes discomfort for the tops of the feet, place a small rolled blanket under them. If you like, you can place a folded blanket over your heels before sitting down.

SITTING IN A CHAIR

Sit a little away from the backrest so your spine will be straight. If your feet don't easily touch the ground, rest them on a rolled blanket or telephone book. Fold a blanket several times to make a long pad. Experiment with it lying across the knees in any of these poses. By placing the backs of your hands on the support, your elbows will bend more and softness will come into the palms.

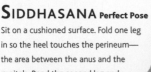

SIDDHASANA Perfect Pose

Sit on a cushioned surface. Fold one leg in so the heel touches the perineum—the area between the anus and the genitals. Bend the second leg and bring the heel of that foot level with the first one. Rest the backs of your hands on your knees.

UJJAYI PRANAYAMA

VICTORIOUS BREATH

Uj comes from the word for "up" and *jaya* means "triumph" or "conquest." Become victorious over any imbalance in the upward-moving prana with Ujjayi breathing. As you grow more comfortable with Ujjayi breathing, use it for the duration of your asana practice.

Ujjayi breathing is a little like drinking air through a straw. The glottis lies in the larynx, near the Adam's apple. It's the part of the throat that closes when you gargle or hold your breath. As the air flows past the partially closed glottis, friction is produced. This friction increases heat in the body, allowing it to stretch more than it otherwise would during yoga asana practice. Ujjayi breathing thins the breath, giving control over the flow of air into the lungs so that the breath becomes steadier, deeper, and longer. More oxygen is made available, enhancing the purification and nourishment of each and every cell.

1. Sit in your meditative position. Breathe in through the nose and out through the mouth. Each time you exhale, make a long "haaaa" sound through your mouth, as if you were trying to fog up a mirror.

2. After several cycles, close your mouth midway through an exhalation, but continue to make the "haaaa" with your lips together. It will become a soft sound like a "hm" that you can feel in the back of the throat. To check if you've got it, cover your ears with your palms and listen to the internal throaty sound. It will sound like the ocean.

3. Now bring it into the inhalation. Open your mouth again and make this "haaaa" sound as you suck in the air. Close your mouth midway through to experience the soft, throaty friction again. When you feel you have got it, cover your ears to check the ocean-like quality of the sound.

4. Now you are ready for the continuous internal "hm" breathing with your mouth closed. At first, practice Ujjayi for ten to 20 breaths while sitting. Take breaks to return to your natural breath whenever you need. This breath is soft in nature and volume.

The sound provides a point of focus for your internalized awareness. It's not necessary to breathe loudly or aggressively. While the sound produced is audible to someone close by, it's not necessary to fill the whole room. Measure the quality of your Ujjayi breathing, not by volume, but by length and steadiness. Bring your awareness to the constancy that this breath gives you. There should be no surges in the breath. It should be clean, even, and pleasant. Each inhalation extends in a long, fluid way to fill the lungs completely. Likewise, the flow of air through your nostrils is slow and steady for the entire duration of the exhalation.

EXPLORE

A few rounds of Ujjayi will center you whenever you like. You can practice it whenever you are tense, or while out walking. Using Ujjayi breathing during your yoga asana practice will focus your mind.

DISCOVERING THE BREATH

BREATHING IN ALL DIRECTIONS

This exercise is usually done with a partner, but can also be done alone. Lightly place your own hands where a partner's hands would be. Then let your shoulders slide up and elbows fall down toward the floor as you curl your palms around your sides. Alternatively, you can hug yourself, placing your hands below your armpits. Finally, let your elbows and shoulders be as heavy and relaxed as possible, as you place your hands on your back ribs. Helpers can direct their breath to the same areas as their partner. You may find that you both begin to breathe in time.

BREATHING INTO THE FRONT

1. Lie on your back with your knees bent and feet flat on the floor. With feet wider than hips, lean your knees together. Helpers need to be sitting perfectly comfortably so they can hold the position for the duration. Any tension will spill over to their partner. Your helper places one palm over your navel and the other high up on the chest, little finger just below the notch at the base of the throat, using a light touch to increase awareness. Have your partner read the instructions, with generous pauses after each sentence to allow you to explore.

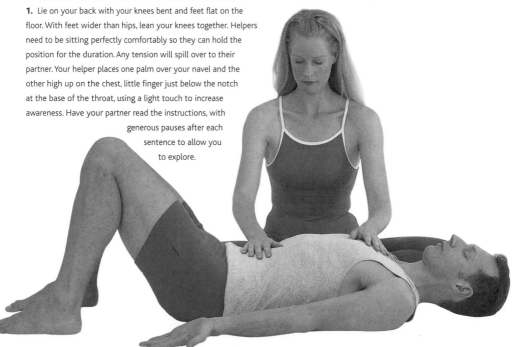

2. Close your eyes. Observe how your body moves with each inhalation. Which part of your body moves first? Can you feel where the breath originates? What happens next? Observe the sequence of movement. What happens to the lower and upper abdomen? How does the ribcage alter? And the chest? Which part feels like it expands more? Let the breath move you. What happens to the shoulders, the throat? Is there any tightness or constriction there? What about the face and nostrils?

3. Now turn your attention to the out breath. From where does your exhalation begin? Where does your exhalation end? Are the movements in the torso as clearly demarcated as in your inhalation? There is a yielding quality to the exhalation, a slow release as the body softens down into the floor. Can you feel a sort of consolidation in toward the center of your torso as you exhale? Could it be that the exhalation ends prematurely? Can you extend the exhalation by being patient and not rushing on to the next breath?

Breathing into the Sides

1. Maintain the quiet stillness as your partner changes position to hold the side ribs, cupping just under the armpits. Observe the horizontal expansion of the ribs on the inhalation, the outward and upward movement each time you draw air in. If you don't feel much movement, exhale more fully so that the inhalation naturally deepens. Observe how each exhalation brings a downward and inward movement.

2. Now pay attention to the timing of these movements in relation to your abdomen and chest. As you inhale, you might find the abdomen expands first, then the side ribs move up and out and, finally, the upper chest expands. If this movement is difficult to isolate, then you should momentarily try to deepen your breathing so that you can discover your particular pattern. What is your pattern of breathing out? Can you isolate the order of movement of the abdomen, side ribs, and chest, or do they seem to run together?

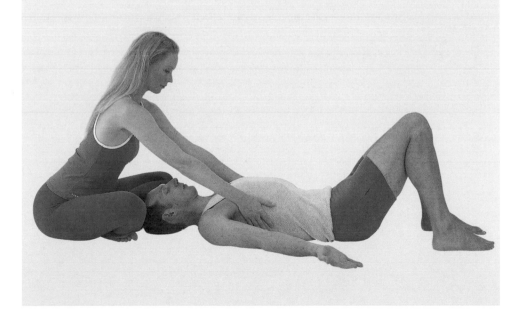

BREATHING INTO THE BACK

1. Keeping your mental focus, kneel and fold forward into Child Pose. You need to be completely comfortable, so for modifications of the posture *see* page 23. Your partner places his or her hands just below your shoulder blades, fingers wrapping around the sides.

2. Take your breath to the back of your body. Mentally direct the air into your partner's hands. As if you had little balloons under your partner's hands, feel your inhalation "puff" out against them. Have patience as you wait for the movement to come. Many people find this rather difficult, and developing this awareness may take several practices.

3. In the beginning, you might find it helpful to limit your breathing into the front of the torso by slightly holding in the part of the abdomen below the navel. Visualize the breath moving into the back of the body. In addition, have your partner press in slightly during your exhalation to remind you where to expand to on the inhalation. Once you begin to get a feeling for it, you will feel the whole back come alive. It opens and blossoms with each inhalation, before softening down on each exhalation.

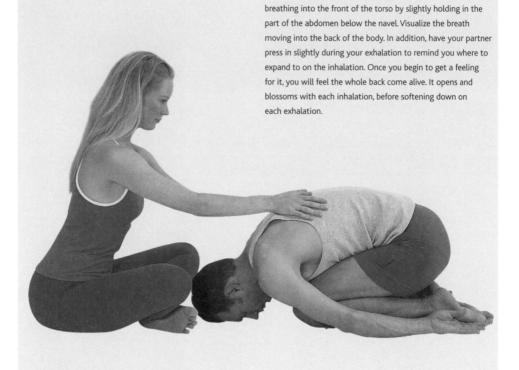

EXPLORE

Once you are able to isolate breathing into the back, you can take the breath up the spine. Each time you inhale, visualize the inhalation starting at the base of the spine and moving all the way up towards the head. Each inhalation energizes the spine, and each exhalation consolidates that energy, filling the body with prana.

BHRAMARI HUMMING BEE BREATH

48

Making sounds is a great way to bring constancy to the breath. It also lengthens the exhalation, which will naturally deepen the inhalation and encourage a slow, rhythmic breath. Don't be shy of making a sound out loud. The sound provides a point of focus for the mind. As the *Hatha Yoga Pradipika* states, "By this practice one becomes lord of the yogis and the mind is absorbed in bliss." Lose yourself in the vibrations and simply enjoy the soothing effect of Bhramari on the mind.

1. Sit comfortably erect or lie with your knees bent. Have your mouth closed, jaw relaxed, and the teeth slightly apart. Pressing your tongue lightly to the roof of the mouth will create a slight tension and turn the simple humming more into a beelike droning.

2. Inhale fully, then exhale while making a humming sound. The vocal cords keep just a small amount of tension so the pitch is low. The constancy of the exhalation keeps the sound uniform. The vibration comes from the soft palate at the top of the back of the mouth. Widen the inside of the mouth to increase the resonance in the nasal cavity. Hone your awareness of the vibration to expand it to the throat, to the top of the head, and eventually to the rest of the body. Practice Bhramari for two minutes and build to five. Afterward, sit or lie quietly with eyes closed to enjoy the aftereffects. Should you experience dizziness or tingling, or should your mind become agitated, switch to simple breathing.

3. Another position for practice is sitting on a blanket with your knees bent in front of you. Place your elbows on your knees so that you can easily cover your eyes with your hands and the flap over your earholes with your thumbs. Become absorbed in the sound that seems to fill the skull.

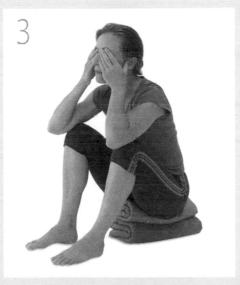

3

EXPLORE

Don't let stress creep in during any breathing exercise. Trying "too hard" changes the lungs, diaphragm, and nervous system, which in turn will adversely affect your body and mind. Evenness in the breath will lead to evenness of temperament.

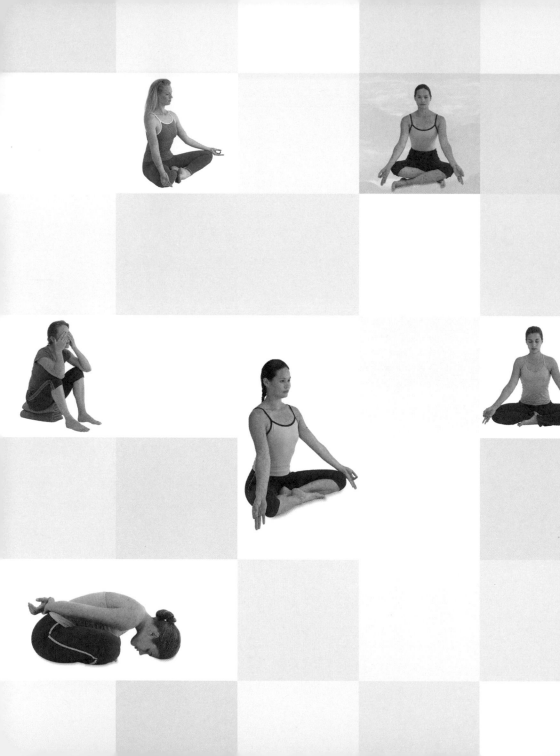

MEDITATION

MEDITATION

Gazing at the sun with wide-open eyes blinds the vision. If you don't stare at it directly, but instead look away a little, you can get a sense of it. Meditation is like that. A change of focus reduces the glare of superfluous distractions and helps us see past the false perceptions to contact the peace and happiness that reside within.

Meditation quietens the mind. Of the eight limbs of Yoga, it is placed seventh, close to the culmination of the state of yoga—the cessation of all the fluctuations of the thoughts. During meditation, we open up the space between the end of one thought and the beginning of the new one.

Meditators do not tune out life's challenges. Rather, they gain greater insight into their perceptions and their response to stressful situations. As the brain patterns merge into the "theta state"—deeper than sleep—the meditator experiences a state of restful alertness: fully conscious and aware. In meditation we practice being the observer, not the doer. We observe our thoughts and remain detached, without altering the thought patterns at all. Remaining neutral toward our thoughts means that we do not lend them energy to disturb the mind. Whereas before you might have been seeing yourself and the world in a dusty mirror, meditation helps to wipe the mirror clean for new perceptions and true reflections.

STUDIES—BLOOD PRESSURE

Many studies have been done on meditation, particularly Transcendental Meditation (TM), which involves meditation using a mantra for 20 minutes, twice a day. A study made in 1996 on hypertensive African-Americans in California found that TM significantly lowered blood pressure—more than did any other relaxation technique or education and lifestyle changes. Those who practiced TM for three months saw an average reduction of ten to 12 points in systolic blood pressure and six to eight points in diastolic pressure (similar results to those of antihypertensive drugs). Through meditation, participants had decreased their risk of heart attack by 11 percent, and stroke by 8–15 percent.

STRESS AND RELATED DISEASES

Researchers at Harvard Medical School used MRI technology to monitor brain activity on meditators. They found that meditation activates the sections of the brain in charge of the autonomic nervous system. This governs the functions in our bodies that we can't control, such as digestion and blood pressure. As these functions are often compromised by stress, it could mean that by lessening the adrenaline surges that arise as a response to stress, meditation would decrease stress-related conditions, such as hypertension, heart disease, asthma, insomnia, digestive problems, and so on.

A study on stress levels was published in the *American Journal of Health Promotion*. Sixty-two people who reported abnormally high levels of stress participated. Twenty-seven people were the control group. Thirty-five underwent 28 hours of "mindfulness training" involving meditation, yoga postures, and stress-relief techniques over two months. After three months, the mindfulness trainees reported a 54 percent drop in psychological distress, as well as a 46 percent reduction in medical symptoms. The control group reported no improvement in psychological symptoms and a slight increase in medical complaints.

HEALING

The word "meditation" comes from the Latin root *meditor*, which literally means "healing," and meditation has been found to reduce costs in health care. In Canada, researchers tracked a group of 677 people enrolled in a health insurance program. After learning TM, their health care payments were reduced by 5–7 percent cumulatively every year. After seven years, health costs had been cut by almost 50 percent. Another study of health insurance statistics was published in *Psychosomatic Medicine*. It studied more than 2,000 people practicing TM over a five-year period. It found they had 50 percent fewer doctors' visits and fewer than half the hospitalizations of other groups of similar age, profession, and insurance coverage. Meditators had fewer incidents of illness in 17 categories, including 87 percent fewer hospitalizations for heart disease and 55 percent fewer for cancer.

INTELLIGENCE

A study published in the *British Journal of Personal and Individual Differences* showed that students practicing Transcendental Meditation increased their IQ by five points in two years and by nine points in four years.

AGING

Meditation has even been found to slow aging. A study in *The International Journal of Neuroscience* found that a group of 50-year-olds who were practicing Transcendental Meditation for over five

years showed a 12-year decrease in "biological age" as compared with controls. And in the words of one old-timer, "Meditators grow older but they don't necessarily have to grow old."

An ancient healer said, "Man is ill, because he is never still." In India, teachers often refer to our monkey-like minds, which flit around randomly. The Vedas, the earliest known compilations of Indian spiritual writings, say the mind is harder to control than the wind. Achieving the cessation of thought patterns is certainly a tall order, but don't be disheartened. Even if you never arrive at this point, enormous benefits can be derived along the path. The Latin root word *meditor* comes from the Sanskrit *madha*, meaning "wisdom." Meditators feel that meditation improves their quality of life and gives them a sense of the inner peace that is at the core of all of us. This superconscious state allows us to re-center. We tap into a positive universal energy, something greater than ourselves. It gives a wonderful feeling of being completely known—sort of like the feeling you have when your beloved has seen all of you, good and bad, and still loves you. Meditation is a source of great inner strength and is something wonderful to come home to.

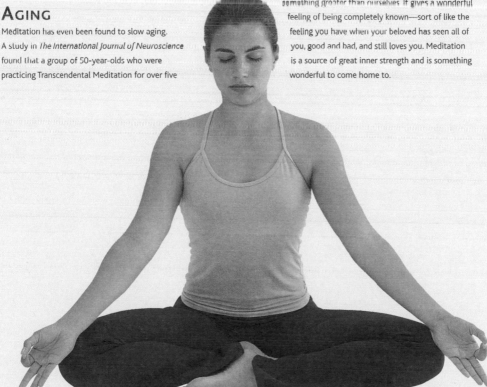

YOGAMUDRASANA SEALING POSE

49

This pose quietens the mind and is a good preparation pose for meditation. Alternatively, you can practice becoming absorbed in the breath (*see* page 134) or Bhramari (*see* page 137).

Sit in Siddhasana (*see* page 132) by first folding your right leg in, then bringing the left heel in front of the right. Grasp your left wrist with your right hand behind your back. Inhale and extend the torso upward, then exhale and fold forward, bringing your forehead to the floor. Rest for at least a minute, observing the breath and the mind. Then, with eyes closed, come up and change sides with the legs and hands before repeating.

For the mind to quieten you need to be physically comfortable. If this seated position does not feel steady and easy, then practice while sitting on the heels. Rest the forehead on a folded blanket if necessary.

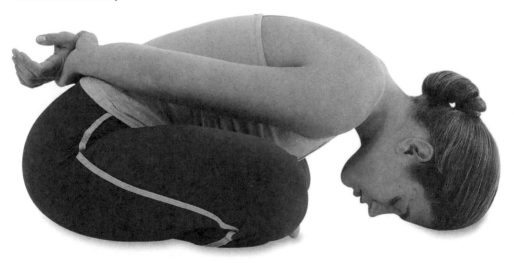

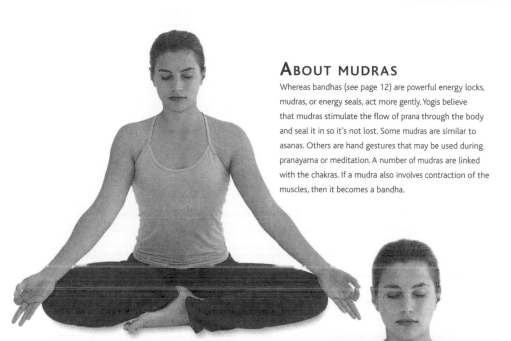

ABOUT MUDRAS

Whereas bandhas (see page 12) are powerful energy locks, mudras, or energy seals, act more gently. Yogis believe that mudras stimulate the flow of prana through the body and seal it in so it's not lost. Some mudras are similar to asanas. Others are hand gestures that may be used during pranayama or meditation. A number of mudras are linked with the chakras. If a mudra also involves contraction of the muscles, then it becomes a bandha.

USEFUL MUDRAS FOR MEDITATION

Mudras influence the subtle bodies and increase receptiveness to higher states of consciousness.

For Gyana Mudra (also called Jnana Mudra) join the tip of the thumb and index finger while keeping the other fingers straight.

For Bhajrava Mudra (Gesture of Shiva), place your right hand on your left. Rest your hands in your lap, with your palms facing up, and let the tips of your thumbs touch.

How to Meditate

A natural time for meditation is at the end of your yoga asana practice, when the body is warm and loose. Otherwise, do a few limbering stretches that release your body and bring you into the present moment. Then follow these six steps.

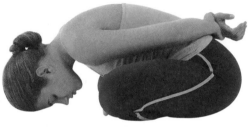

Above: Yogamudrasana.

1. Set the Body

You can practice Yogamudrasana (*see* page 142), Discovering the Breath (*see* page 134), or Bhramari breathing (*see* page 137).

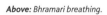

Above: Bhramari breathing.

Right: Discovering the breath.

2. Set the Mind

Decide how long you will sit for. Choose a quiet place and turn off the phone. Cover yourself with a blanket or shawl if necessary. Assume your meditative position. Make sure the back, neck, and head are in line. See the pranayama section (page 128) for suggested sitting positions.

Some people like to offer a personal prayer or chant as a little ritual to carry them into the session. In any case, clarify your intention, reminding yourself of your higher goal and your reason for meditating.

3. Relax the Body

While seated, mentally check in with each part of the body. Start from your toes and relax everything bit by bit up to the crown of your head. Once relaxed, commit to not moving your body any more. Any physical movement only serves to distract.

4. Focus the Mind

The breath is a wonderful tool to deepen concentration. Begin by observing the flow of air through the nostrils. Observe the minute sensations at the nostrils: the cool air as it flows in through the nostrils, and the warmed air that flows out. There is no need to judge your breath or change the way you are breathing. Patiently be aware simply of what is. You are the detached observer. Practicing detachment is useful for the times in life that you are challenged by pain or difficulty. If you like, count your breaths in rounds of ten.

5. Expansion of Consciousness

Steer your thoughts to an attitudinal theme or virtue; a hypergoal such as freedom from attachments, inner peace, or spiritual self-realization.

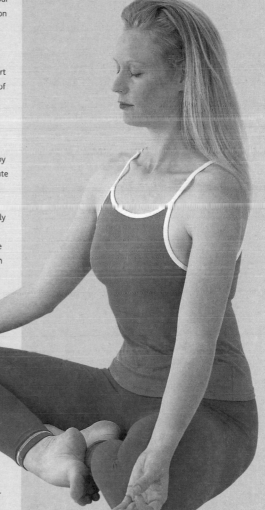

6. Finally

To close, repeat a prayer or use a chant if you find it helpful. When your time for sitting has ended, don't jump up and start racing through your day in an automated way. You have just connected with your inner self with a greater force. Stay mindful and carry this sensation through into your daily life and personal relationships.

MEDITATION TECHNIQUES

Meditation is a deeply personal thing. More than a technique or a practice, meditation is an experience. There is no one way that is better than another. Try out some ways to see what you feel works best for you. After some experimentation, find a technique with which you feel an affinity and stick to it for at least several months.

CHAKRA MEDITATION

By moving your awareness to the appropriate physical spot on the body, you can meditate on a chakra. Each chakra has a seed sound associated with it, which you can use as a mantra. Alternatively, you may choose to meditate on the pure color of the chakra (*see* page 152 for chakra mantras and colors).

Right: Trataka, or steady gazing, will develop into a meditation over time.

TRATAKA Steady Gazing

Trataka is a good practice for dharana, or concentration, the sixth limb of yoga. You may gaze at a lit candle, picture, symbol, or deity to which you feel drawn. Over time, trataka moves from being a concentration exercise to become a meditation.

MANTRA MEDITATION

Many people derive great benefit from using a mantra. *See* page 148 for more information on mantras.

MOVING MEDITATION

Any action performed with mindfulness can be meditative. A walking meditation is useful if you find sitting for long periods very uncomfortable, or if you tend to fall asleep. You might begin sitting, then, when you are ready, stand up. Keep your eyes unfocused, gazing down to the floor. Walk with your awareness on the feet. Feel the sensations in each sole as it rolls down to contact the floor, bears weight, and then peels off the floor to take the next step. Stay keenly focused on the changes in the weight borne by each foot as you slowly walk in a circle. After this walking meditation, sit and continue the meditation.

THEMED MEDITATIONS

Choose a subject on which you would like to expand your awareness, such as love or peace. During breath or mantra meditation you attempt to confine the thoughts to a single subject—the breath or the mantra. In a themed meditation you can expand your consciousness by further refining the focus: from many thoughts around a subject, you can reduce to a single thought on it.

The aim is not to prevent all thought but to attain a one-pointed awareness. Observe the flow of thought, like ripples in a lake, without following them. If you follow a thought that isn't the focus of your meditation, you are lending it the energy to distract yourself. Practice mastery over the mind and gently bring your mind back to your chosen subject. The constant churning of the mind eventually gives way to peacefulness.

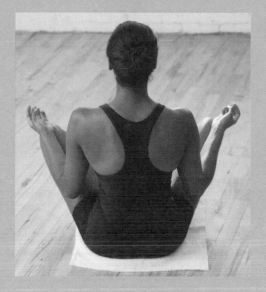

Right: The aim of meditation is not to prevent all thought but to attain a one-pointed awareness.

MORE ON MEDITATION

Set aside a regular time to meditate. Yogis believe the best times of day to meditate are sunrise, noon, sunset, or midnight, but the most important thing is to find a time in your schedule that you know you will be able to stick to. Don't set yourself up for failure by choosing an impossible time. Likewise, decide realistically how long you can dedicate to each meditation. Then keep to it—don't come out of it early. Some people use a timer set to beep gently when the time has elapsed. Traditionally, east- or north-facing positions are considered conducive to spiritual practice.

Sitting perfectly still can become difficult because every physical sensation is magnified. Breathe through itches as they arise. Remind yourself that all things change; these sensations are only transitory, and can provide the energy for better focus. For a busy mind, being mindful—doing nothing except paying attention—gets boring. Instead of inventing things to relieve this boredom, stay with the meditation, accept that you are feeling bored, and make it the subject of your attention for a while.

Although meditation brings people peace, it can also bring to mind other issues. As a process of self-observation, you may be confronted with thoughts or parts of your character that you would prefer not to recognize. Facing certain feelings you are not owning up to can raise your level of anxiety, as if there is nowhere to hide. Although it can be very disturbing, remind yourself that all things change. Becoming aware of your shadow side actually allows you to operate in a different way.

Like your yoga practice, meditation experiences will vary from day to day. Don't classify meditations as "good" or "bad." Perhaps a meditation feels "bad" because it has thrown up something you find uncomfortable. It might feel more difficult but could actually offer you a lot. Try not to become too attached to the highs you experience on your spiritual path. If we cling to these feelings we may miss the point of the exercise, which is a feeling of unity with the universe as a whole. Refrain from judging the highs and lows and simply welcome that experience as part of the unceasing flow of life.

In meditation, we often seek to encourage a detachment from worldly things. While this type of detachment can assist us in objective observation, it does not mean that we should stop caring about what happens to the world. We need to continue interacting in an open-minded and loving way.

MANTRAS AND CHANTING

A mantra is a potent sound that helps harmonize the system, a vibrational force that carries healing. Reciting a mantra or devotional verse in a yogic chant is uplifting and soothing.

MANTRA

A mantra can be a syllable, a word, or a phrase that is generally repeated over and over. Using a mantra provides a point of focus for the mind. A mantra is a positive affirmation: a constant reminder and a way to bring yourself back to base. Reciting a mantra is an exercise in *dharana* (concentration) that can become *dhyana* (meditation).

Many mantras are in the ancient language of Sanskrit. Sanskrit is made up of primordial sounds, and each syllable creates a particular resonance within the body. A Sanskrit mantra is a particular combination of sound vibrations which, when chanted or meditated upon, has a specific effect on the body, mind, and psyche. This resonance assists healing and spiritual elevation. In each repetition a certain energetic vibration is being sent out into the world. For this reason the pronunciation needs to be exact, so if you are not sure, ask a yoga teacher about the correct pronunciation for your mantra.

Though traditionally given by a guru, you can certainly choose your own mantra. It is not necessary to have an exotic-sounding mantra. You may feel more affinity with a mantra in your own language such as peace, love, or faith.

If you would like to use a mantra for meditation, you can begin each session by chanting the mantra aloud and letting the resonance flow through the body. Then, keeping the reverberation, take the volume down to a whisper and, finally, continue your meditation by repeating it mentally.

A mantra is often used at the beginning and end of a yoga class. It can be as simple as chanting *om* three times with the teacher. You can link your mantra practice to work with particular areas of the body and the chakras (*see page 152*). Many people find using a mantra helps in times of stress—even in public places a mantra can be repeated silently. Like an affirmation, it's a helpful reminder to bring you back to base.

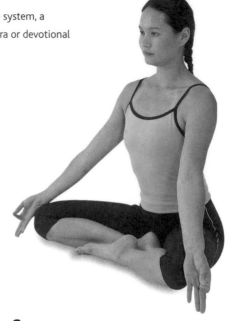

SOME COMMON MANTRAS

Om—This sacred syllable is considered the mother of all sounds. As with other Sanskrit mantras, it is believed that it sets up a special vibration in your body and mind, and this is spread out into the world. It is used by both Hindus and Buddhists. *Om* is composed of the three sounds *A-U-Mmmm* running together. The first "A" sound will resonate more in the belly. The "U" moves the vibration up to the chest cavity. The final long "M" sound is made into a nasal sound so its resonance is felt more in the head.

Om namah shivaya—This is a salutation to the Hindu deity Shiva. Non-Hindus use this mantra, too, intending it to honor the divine in oneself.

Soham—This mantra also honors the divine within. Pronounced *so-hum*, it means "I am the universal self."

Shanti—Means "peace" in Sanskrit.

Om namo bhagavate vasudevaya—Means salutations to the Divine Source, the indweller of all.

CHANTING

Though some adults feel shy about making sounds out loud, chanting is really perfectly natural. Let go of worrying about how good or bad you sound. Chanting is not like singing but more like reciting. The purpose is not to have the most beautiful voice, but rather to feel the sound resonate through the body.

The devotional path of yoga is called Bhakti yoga where God or God's representative spiritual teacher is worshipped. In Bhakti yoga, spiritual verses are chanted with fervent devotion. There is a sense of connection to something greater than the self, as the heart center opens up to a crescendo of universal love. Then the emotions are settled down to stabilize once

more. This climax and settling of the emotions is similar to a heartbroken person crying out a song about lost love. When the emotions are relived in a small way, then left to settle, it's very healing on the emotional sphere.

Even if you don't consider yourself religious, chanting can be a worthwhile and fulfilling experience. A chanting session is incredibly soothing. It feels like a balm for the brain. It seems to wipe away all the usual preoccupations, so it's like taking an instant mental vacation. In addition, it clarifies your intentions and is uplifting for the heart. If you are not comfortable with a chant to God, you may feel more comfortable interpreting it as being a chant to the light you carry within. If you ask around, you may find a chanting group in your area.

CHANTS TO START AND FINISH YOUR YOGA PRACTICE

Om asathoma sadgamaya
Thamasoma Jyotirgamaya
Mrithyorma Amrithangamaya
Om Shanti Shanti Shanti

Om Lead me from the unreal to the real
From darkness to light
From the predicament of death to immortality
Om peace, peace, peace

Om
Swasthi praja bhyah pari pala yantam
Nya yena margena mahi mahi shaha
Go brahmanebhyaha shubhamastu nityam
Lokaa samastha sukhino bhavantu
Om

Om
Let prosperity be glorified
Let rulers rule the world with law and justice
Let divinity and wisdom be protected
Let people of the world be happy and prosperous
Om

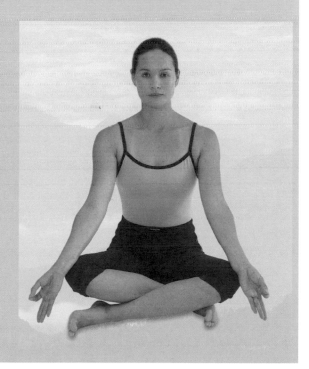

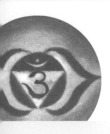

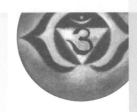

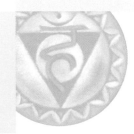

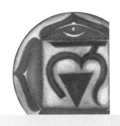

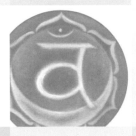

THE KUNDALINI PATH

CHAKRAS

Hatha yoga exercises focus on the vertebral column and work not only on the physical body but also on the subtle bodies. The twisting, lengthening, and bending forward, backward, and sideways of hatha yoga aim to awaken and balance the subtle energies.

According to the yogic tradition, there are many thousands of "nadis"—energy meridians—in our bodies. The largest one is called the Sushumna nadi. It is not recognized by Western anatomy but it follows a nervous pathway, running from the perineum up the length of the vertebral column.

Yogis speak of a reservoir of energy known as the *kundalini,* which resides in the body. Literally translated as "she who is coiled," the kundalini force is likened to a serpent lying dormant at the base of the spine. Yoga exercises seek to undo any energy blockages of the spine, and purify the body and mind to clear the way for this cosmic power to rise. Another way to clear the kundalini path is to work with the chakras.

The word *chakra* means "wheel" in Sanskrit. A chakra, like a wheel or vortex, is an area of increased energy (prana). As a center of energy, a chakra can exist anywhere in the body, though we tend to recognize seven main ones located at various levels up the spine. It is said that the chakras act as transformers. As each chakra has a related nerve and endocrine plexus, they are believed to channel the pranic energy into the physical body at the points of the chakras. It is thought that when all the chakras are fully functioning, the kundalini power can move unimpeded up the body's central energy channel from the base of the spine to the crown of the head. As the kundalini "serpent" uncoils and rises, it enlivens each chakra in turn. When it reaches the top chakra, it is said that a change of consciousness occurs, special psychic powers are obtained, and liberation of the soul (the ultimate goal of yoga) is attained.

Each of these seven reservoirs of energy has its own physical, emotional, and spiritual effects. The lower chakras, from the base of the spine to the solar plexus, are considered to be more physical than the chakras located from the heart to the crown of the head. Many people choose to focus their work on the higher chakras, believing them to be more "spiritual" than the more earthy lower ones. However, like building a house, each level needs to be supported by a solid base below it. The grounding forces of the lower chakras provide the vital steady foundation for balanced spiritual exploration. Should a chakra be out of balance, yoga can help stimulate the less active chakras and move energy along from areas where it is congested, therefore balancing the system. Knowledge of the chakras allows us to understand ourselves a little more; yoga postures are tools with which to facilitate transformation.

1 MULADHARA CHAKRA—ROOT CHAKRA

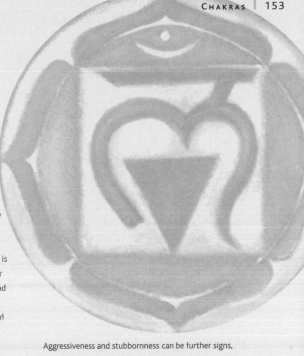

Location

The base of the spine is the home of the first chakra. The related organs are the organs of elimination and excretion—the lungs, skin, kidneys, large intestine, and rectum.

Expression

The root chakra governs your connection to the earth and how "rooted" you feel. It deals with your material and monetary existence. It is the chakra that is concerned with getting your basic needs met—like obtaining food, shelter, and even love. It is very involved with how stable you feel emotionally and in your physical setup. The root chakra is expressed in your strength and stamina. It gives you the drive to get up and go to work in the morning. It allows you to focus, be disciplined, stay healthy, and be aware of your limits.

The root chakra must be balanced as a foundation to balancing the other chakras or your progression will be without roots and stability. When the muladhara chakra is out of balance, it may cause problems of the lower abdominal area, such as constipation, diarrhea, hemorrhoids, kidney problems, sciatica, and back pain.

As the base chakra has such a grounding force, the psychological impact of imbalance at the level of this chakra can swing from being too grounded to not being grounded enough. A lack of grounding could cause you to live in a fantasy world and feel off-center. You could experience difficulty focusing, or find that you go out of control easily. You may find it hard to contain your feelings. On the other hand there may be too much holding on: for example, if you are excessively materialistic or unable to let go of things emotionally. It might manifest itself in being overly controlling and trying to keep a hold over others.

The muladhara chakra is the driving force behind the energy to work. When this chakra is not in balance, you could become overly attached to your work, leading to a workaholic lifestyle. Another manifestation could be diminished creative power, which will interfere with your ability to enjoy life and prevent you from opening up to feelings of joy and happiness.

Aggressiveness and stubbornness can be further signs, as can a tendency toward selfishness, creating material and emotional possessiveness. An imbalance in the root chakra can make you self-serving and self-centered. When your survival is threatened, you feel afraid. This fear can be immobilizing and ultimately prevent you from achieving your goals. The root chakra is awakened when you confront your fears.

When the root chakra is functioning well, there will be good general health for the related organs, like the kidneys and bowel. The adrenal glands, involved in the response to stress, will be healthy, not exhausted from chronic overstimulation. There will be a cheerful, fearless, and courageous attitude. A balanced base chakra brings self-confidence, enthusiasm, a strong will to live, and a clear sense of identity. Trust in others comes easily.

You will have a good perspective on life and be able to stay in touch with the greater scheme of things. You will be able to detach from an overemphasis on the importance of material possessions. There will be a healthy attitude to work. While you will remain focused, you will not be so attached to your work that you ignore other parts of your life. You will approach your work and challenges with enthusiasm and joy. With this attitude, material success can come to you more easily.

2 SVADHISTHANA CHAKRA—SEXUAL CHAKRA

Location

The second chakra is located at the lower abdomen between the navel and the genitals. The second chakra governs the organs of the lower abdominal area, such as those of the urinary and reproductive systems.

Expression

Its location is a clue that the second chakra is involved with sexuality, relationships, and creativity. The svadhisthana chakra governs our nurturing abilities and our sensation and pleasure focus. It is also highly involved in relationships, and this includes your relationship with yourself.

Change is an inescapable fact of life. Without change, there is no growth, no movement, no life. The sexual chakra is connected with change and how you deal with it. A well-balanced second chakra allows you to go with the flow and alter your path as necessary.

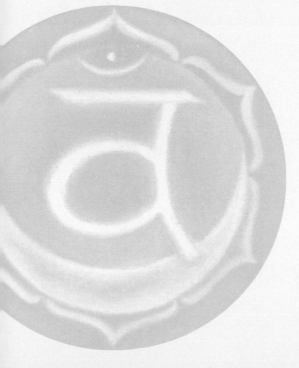

If you have an imbalance in this chakra, it could affect the urinary, reproductive, and circulatory systems. Impotence, sexually transmitted diseases, and bladder problems could be signs that the second chakra needs some attention.

People who have an unbalanced sexual chakra have difficulty with giving or receiving materially or emotionally. Obesity can be a result of a lack of balance between giving and receiving. An overweight person who is consuming more calories than they are using is taking more than they are giving. The second chakra helps with assimilation of knowledge. On the mental level, receiving is linked with the integration of knowledge as the brain takes in and stores information.

Feelings of guilt, anxiety, unpredictability, and clinging on can be an indication of an unbalanced second chakra. Some people may have difficulty separating their own feelings from those of others. General low energy or lack of creativity can also be connected to this chakra. Sexual desire may be too little or too much. Flirting outrageously or using sex as a way to gain attention are further signs that the chakra is off balance. A person may become trapped in an unhealthy pattern of seeking excessive sensual pleasure.

A well-balanced second chakra gives a high level of general vitality. The lower abdominal, urinary, and reproductive systems will be healthy. If this chakra is balanced, you will be outgoing, patient, and have a good sense of humor. You will be comfortable with your sexuality and content with yourself. You find it easy to be positive and enjoy life.

A main force of this chakra governs the attraction of opposites. There is an unceasing dance between dualities. Movement is created and you can easily go with the flow of life. At the same time, you have intellectual ideas about the world and how your desires and emotions fit in it.

Creative problem-solving and the ability to work creatively with others will come easily. Even if other people have different ideas than you do, you are able to work out a complementary path. Instead of forming obstacles, the different approaches and attitudes of others enrich your life and allow you to develop and grow.

3 MANIPURA CHAKRA— SOLAR PLEXUS

Location

The third chakra is situated between the bottom of the breastbone and the navel. It controls the digestive system and related organs, including the liver, stomach, gall bladder, pancreas, spleen, and the organs of excretion.

Expression

Through its closeness to the digestive system, this third chakra is involved in the production and storage of energy—the same energy that allows us to live our lives effectively. The manipura chakra relates to our emotions, actions, power, and will. It helps us recognize that, with effort and action, we can achieve what we want.

The solar plexus center links to your level of comfort with power, and this includes your sense of personal power. Your power comes through being able to bring things together. Rather than seeing things as separate and unrelated, and subdividing them, you are able to find the power in unification. A balanced third chakra helps you develop a healthy will and autonomy. When unbalanced, you may feel powerless, have lower self-esteem, and be more easily swayed by the opinions of those around you.

If your third chakra is not in balance, you can experience uncontrolled extreme emotions, such as violent passions, jealousies, anger, and frustration, and they can then turn into doubts, fears, and confusion. There may be a tendency to try to manipulate others. Obsessive characteristics or a tendency to an addictive personality might appear.

Failure to learn to assert your own autonomy can cause you to feel powerless or victimized. With an unbalanced third chakra, you risk running out of emotional steam. Apathy and lethargy cause your energy to turn in on itself and make you want to withdraw from life. You can become overly critical of yourself, causing you to lose the ability to connect and be nourished by your surroundings. Low self-esteem makes you doubt yourself, and you can suffer self-recrimination.

There can also be an imbalance of fiery energy. This may manifest itself as feeling hot, avoiding spicy foods, wanting cold drinks, sweating easily, or being quick-tempered. Too little fire, on the other hand, can cause you to feel cold, crave hot, spicy foods and hot drinks, or feel slow and lethargic. Any of the related organs might show symptoms. Internally, ulcers, upset stomach, diabetes, hypoglycemia, or even alcoholism, and, externally, a tight, hard belly, large potbelly, or a sunken diaphragm, may all indicate an imbalance.

A well-balanced manipura chakra gives a great deal of energy, which might show up as having a warm body and fast metabolism. This energy brings an enthusiasm for work, play, development, and transformation in your life. You will feel bright and extroverted and have clear thinking.

You will have a constructive use of power and it will be directed inward, toward the self, instead of being wielded over others. This internal willpower creates proactive, assertive, and confident qualities. Your self-esteem is at a healthy level and there will be a drive toward a consciously controlled positive change, as opposed to passively waiting or wishing for something great to happen. You will be self-motivated and self-accepting. You will be naturally aware of your social responsibility and will approach things from a social perspective. You aren't tempted to abuse your power to manipulate others. Your power is used to bring people and things together, rather than to drive them apart. A balanced manipura chakra produces an inner strength, allowing you to perform actions with ease and grace.

4 ANAHATA CHAKRA—HEART CENTER

Location

Located at the center of the chest, the anahata chakra corresponds to love in the pure, unconditional sense. It encompasses the love of nature and the love of all humanity.

Expression

Physically, the anahata chakra relates to the heart, the circulatory and respiratory systems, the breasts, chest, and shoulders. The fourth chakra brings together the forces of the first three chakras. The first chakra is about solidity and stability, the second governs change and movement, while the third brings into play acceptance and the forces of the will. When these forces come together, they can then be transformed into energies to achieve higher goals. The heart center is the point of transition between the more grounding lower chakras and the higher, spiritual ones.

The heart chakra deals with social awareness, love, and openness, a sense of devotion, peace, forgiveness, acceptance, kindness, and joy. While the second chakra has a unifying force that is oriented more toward objects or people, the unifying force of the heart chakra is experienced more as a state of being. It is less involved with sexuality, less materialistic, and more conceptual. It deals with the union and harmonious integration of the self into larger social groups without any loss of true sense of self. The force of the anahata chakra allows us to break out of the limitations of our ego. In transcending the ego we can grow toward something deep and strong. It loosens our boundaries as we experience the joy of love.

Physically, an imbalance in the fourth chakra could result in heart conditions, including high blood pressure, and could cause respiratory conditions, asthma, and arthritis of the arms. Emotionally, you might tend toward feeling a conditional type of love. Perhaps you expect something in return for giving your love, or you could confuse love and sex. You may impose your will over others, and tend to be manipulative. On the other hand, you might be overly selfless, often finding yourself in the role of martyr. An imbalance might lead to a lack of sensitivity, arrogance, selfishness, or feelings of sadness or depression.

When the heart chakra is in balance, the related organs and systems will be healthy. There is a sense of connection with all life, which gives peace, joy, and feelings of unconditional love for all beings. Your relationships will be more balanced and harmonious. Your emotions will be free but not unstable, and they can be clearly and spontaneously expressed. You will be open, willing and able to live without fear of vulnerability. There will be a good balance between the material things in life and your emotions. Because the heart center has an integrative force, helping us overcome dualities, and because love is the ultimate healing energy, the heart chakra is the center for healing.

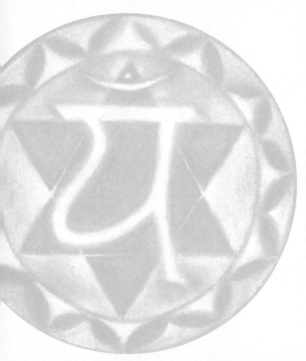

5 VISUDDHA CHAKRA—THROAT CENTER

Location

Located level with the base of the throat, the fifth chakra is linked to communication and expression.

Expression

As its physical location may suggest, the visuddha chakra corresponds to the neck and organs of the neck, including the voice box and airway in the throat. As the related glands are the thyroid and parathyroid glands, the metabolism of the whole body is affected by the fifth chakra.

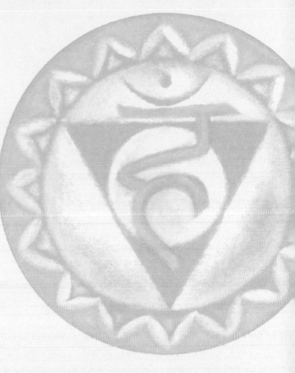

The throat chakra is involved in the verbal expression of all the thoughts and feelings encompassed by the lower chakras. It affects our speech and how we express ourselves. It is linked to truth and honesty. This center connects our feelings and intuition with our thoughts, making them enter our consciousness and enabling us to act on them. The throat chakra helps form our future. A need or desire is more easily met once it is expressed, so in a way, we shape our own futures with verbal communication. Like the second chakra, this fifth chakra is strongly linked to creativity: the formation of speech, communication, and expression make up an inherently creative process. The throat chakra moves away from the physicality of the chakras below. Its boundaries are more fluid and less physical, being involved in such things as the sharing of information and ideas.

Problems with the throat chakra can show up physically in sore throats, loss of voice, and neck or throat conditions. An over- or underactive thyroid, headaches from neck muscle tension, insomnia, flu, and even cancer could be manifestations of an imbalance in this center. Any difficulty in expression or communication indicates an imbalance of the fifth chakra. You may hold back, either in voicing your opinion or showing your thoughts or feelings. On the other hand, you may dominate conversations and discussions. Perhaps you have difficulty expressing your needs or having them met. You could be critical, tactless, deceitful, judgmental, or harsh-voiced, or may suffer from false pride.

When the throat chakra is in balance, the throat area will be physically healthy. You have effective expression and clear communication of your feelings and ideas, and it can show in your voice, making it clear and pleasant to the ear. Creativity, maturity, and inspiration help you deal with yourself and others in an honest, compassionate, and tactful way. You can make clear assessments without judging others. Verbal expression is made possible by vibrational rhythms, and the throat chakra is linked to rhythm and the pace at which we lead our lives. You will be able to conduct your life at a regular, easy pace, rather than losing yourself in a hectic and destructive lifestyle. A balanced fifth chakra gives you a sense of serenity and devotion.

6 AJNA CHAKRA—THIRD EYE CENTER

Location

Located between and just above the eyebrows, the sixth chakra is like a third eye, said to be the seat of wisdom.

Expression

The sixth chakra is linked to the brain and nervous system. The ears, nose, eyes, and sinuses relate to it. Lastly, the hormonal system is affected by the sixth chakra through the wide-reaching effects of the pituitary gland in the brain. The information-gathering capability of our sense of sight is very powerful. With a single glance we can take on board an enormous amount of information. Taking our ability to "see" and assess situations farther, the sixth chakra becomes involved in the capacity for intuition, imagination, visualization, and even clairvoyance. This intuition is the link between our intellectual and psychic abilities. Being guided from within lies beyond the part of the mind telling us we can't do something and the part telling us we can. Intuition is a line to a force greater than ourselves. Physically, an imbalance in the sixth chakra may manifest in headaches or eye, ear, nose, and sinus conditions. Hormonal imbalances, insomnia, and nervous disorders may appear. Depression may arise. The third eye center is linked to the hormonal glands of the brain, and therefore to levels of the neurotransmitter serotonin, depletion of which has been linked to depression.

On another level, depression might come from having lost touch with your essentially creative self—a lack of ability to use and flow with your creativity. When the sixth chakra is out of balance, you can have problems focusing and concentrating and may feel confused and negative. A lack of direction and intellectual stagnation can be experienced. So many people spend many hours a week in a job that doesn't enhance their life. We need to be enriched by what we do. Make sure your work is in harmony with your beliefs. The sixth chakra can help us determine what will enrich us. Your yoga asana practice is useful as it is a journey on the emotional and intellectual level, which opens you up to listen to your intuitive self and the special language of your body: posture, holding patterns, disease, well-being.

When the third eye chakra is in balance, you will be able to observe thoughts and feelings without becoming overly attached to them. You have a good level of direction, devotion, and high ideals. You are imaginative and carry within yourself a sense of oneness, a feeling of unity. This sense of integration allows you to overcome anxiety. When the ajna chakra is fully awakened, you experience a mastery of the self, known as self-realization.

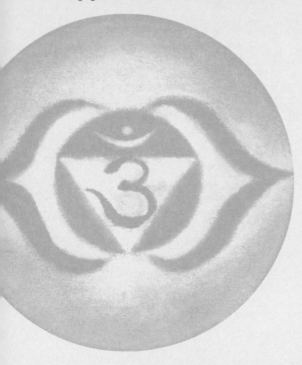

7 SAHASRARA CHAKRA—CROWN CENTER

Location

The crown chakra is located at the top of the head, at the "soft spot" that is the anterior fontanel.

Expression

The brain, the whole nervous system, and the pineal gland are in the realm of the crown chakra. The root chakra and the crown chakras have opposite forces. While the root chakra acts as the entry point of human life, the crown acts as an exit point. The crown chakra deals with transcending materialism and letting go of physical attachments. The search for meaning—that all things are part of a larger structure—brings us closer to unity. The seventh chakra gives us a coherent sense of meaning. It relates to the highest state of consciousness. It deals with spiritual enlightenment, self-realization, and God-consciousness. The crown chakra is very important because it is the point where the liberation of the soul arrives. When the sahasrara chakra is fully awakened, there is a fusion of the seven chakras and the experience of boundlessness. At this level of consciousness, there is an awareness of a higher or deeper order that integrates and unifies. It reminds us that, even though the body is finite, the soul is infinite.

Physically, cerebral tumors and increased pressure in the skull can be an indication of an imbalance in the crown center. There could be psychological symptoms like psychoses or neuroses or depression. Insomnia may occur due to the crown chakra's link with the pineal gland, which produces melatonin: vital for healthy sleep. It is also linked to Seasonal Affective Disorder (SAD), sufferers from which feel down and depressed during colder seasons of less daylight. Emotionally, you may also experience a sense of isolation from the world. There can be a loss of direction, low energy levels, fatigue, and a tendency toward having a "closed mind." When your crown chakra is in balance, you will feel a sense of unity with others without suffering a loss of your individuality. You will pay well-focused attention to them. There is no distortion, but rather a knowledge born of wisdom or enlightenment. You will follow your own ethical ideals and not be overly influenced by outside forces or the opinions of others.

CHAKRAS AT A GLANCE

	Chakra	Color	Element	Relates to	Element	Mantra
	Muladhara	Red	Ruby	Stability, Survival, Basic Needs	Earth	Lam
	Svadhisthana	Orange	Amber	Creativity, Sexuality, Relationships	Water	Vam
	Manipura	Yellow	Gold	Power, Will, Action	Fire	Ram
	Anahata	Green	Emerald	Unconditional Love, Self-Healing, Joy	Air	Yam
	Visuddha	Sky Blue	Sapphire	Communication, Self-Expression, Truth	Ether	Ham
	Ajna	Indigo	Diamond	Intuition, Wisdom	Pure Essence	Om
	Sahasrara	Violet	Amethyst	Spiritual Illumination, The Bliss State	Boundlessness	(no mantra)

Chakra	Balancing the Chakras—General	Meditation	Affirmation	Asanas
Muladhara	Get enough sleep every day and rest when you are tired. Massage is grounding and brings you back to body sensations. Foot massage is good. Eat regularly. Don't skip meals.	You can meditate using the seed mantra for this chakra, Lam.	A useful affirmation for this chakra is to repeat in your mind or out loud about ten times, several times a day: "I stand firmly in my life in a loving and imaginative way."	All the standing postures help balance the root chakra. Tadasana Virabhadrasana I, II, III Garudasana Paschimottanasana Savasana
Svadhisthana	Massage can help you to let go of old emotions. Rolfing is a form of massage that can release memories from body tissue. It is deep and can be cathartic. But there are also gentler forms of massage that can release emotions for those who prefer a softer approach. Pranayama can help in letting go of emotions, especially with long exhalations.	You can meditate on the seed sound, Vam.	"I am open to the world and flow easily with changes in my life."	Trikonasana Pavritta Trikonasana Ardha Baddha Padma Paschimottanasana Baddha Konasana Paschimottanasana
Manipura	Jogging and power walking overcome sluggishness. Stomach crunches tone the area. Laughing or physical exercise help release suppressed emotions. Let go of emotional attachments that aren't helping you. Ask yourself what is running smoothly and enjoyably in your life right now. How can you use your will and less effort to achieve your goals?	You can meditate on empowerment or use the seed mantra, Ram.	"I move toward my goals smoothly and enjoyably."	Twists, back arches, and forward stretches will assist the solar plexus chakra. Pavritta Trikonasana Ustrasana Jathara Parivartanasana Paschimottanasana Purvottanasana Balasana

Chakra	Balancing the Chakras—General	Meditation	Affirmation	Asanas
Anahata	An exercise to open the heart chakra is to sit in a crowded place. Choose a person on who, to focus your mind. While you sit relaxed and breathing deeply, take your time in observing their body movements, their face, their eyes, and the way they speak. Put aside judgment. With each inhalation, build compassion for this person within you, but let go on each exhalation.	You can meditate on the seed mantra, Yam	"My heart opens with love for all beings."	Virabhadrasana I Anjaneyasana Matsyasana Ustrasana Urdva Dhanurasana Passive opening twist Balasana
Visudcha	Because this chakra operates on the level of vibration, chanting that works with the vibration of sound has a purifying effect. See the section on mantras (page 148). The breath can be used to calm the nervous system and enhance the quality of the voice, making it fuller, deeper, and clearer. Practice Bhramari and Ujjayi breathing (see pages 137 and 133 respectively).	You can meditate on the seed mantra, Ham, or chant it aloud	"I communicate honestly and directly."	Matsyasana Ustrasana Setu Bandhasana Sarvangasana Halasana Karnapidasana
Ajna	Meditation is key to opening the third eye chakra. Sit in a quiet place and focus on your breathing. Allow your breath to move to the area between and just above the eyebrows. Alternatively, do a color meditation, visualizing in turn each of the colors from the first to seventh chakras. From red, move through orange, yellow, green, blue, indigo, and violet.	The seed sound for this chakra is Om.	"I am open to my inner guidance," or "I follow my inner guidance."	Matsyasana Setu bandhasana Sarvangasana Balasana Sirsasana Yogamudrasana
Sahasrara	To activate the crown chakra, live your life with as much awareness as possible. While this is more easily said than done, you can use breath awareness exercises, meditation, affirmation, and asanas to help you.	Meditation taps into the world of the seventh chakra. There is no seed sound for this chakra, though you could chant the ancient sacred sound, Om.	"My soul is boundless and infinite."	Any meditation pose sitting erect with the back, neck, and head in line is beneficial to working with the crown chakra. Siddhasana Vajarasana Balasana Sirsasana Sasankasana Yogamudrasana

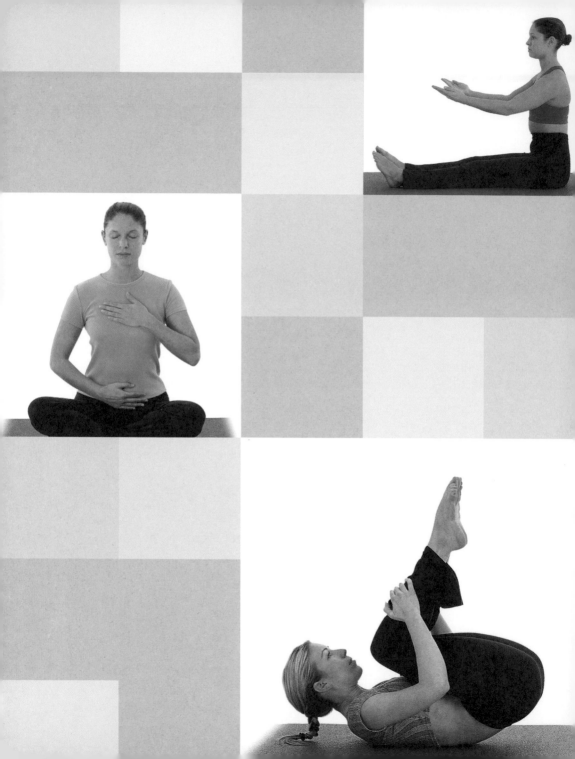

PILATES

INTRODUCTION

The Pilates technique was developed in the early years of the 20th century by a young German who was determined to overcome his physical disabilities and become a fit and healthy individual. His efforts were totally successful, and his methods are not only still used today, but are growing in popularity as the benefits of this gentle form of exercise are recognized.

The technique, consisting of a series of controlled, flowing movements, will not only improve your shape but will also promote flexibility, remedy any postural problems you may have, by realigning your body structure to its natural balance, and allow internal organs to function more efficiently. The primary aim of the exercises is to promote stability in the "core" or "center" of the body—that is, the area around your middle where the muscles that support the spine are located—and in the shoulder girdle and pelvis.

This is not frenetic aerobic exercise, to be carried out mechanically to the thumping rhythm of deafening music: Pilates involves focused concentration and conscious flowing breath. Each movement is carried out with balance and precision, and you maintain a constant connection between mind and body, feeding information between the two. Pilates is a truly holistic approach to physical and mental health and harmony.

Does this sound too good to be true? Are you wondering where the catch is? Well, there isn't one —the only thing you need to bear in mind is that Pilates is not a "quick fix." It takes time and can be tough, especially if you are starting from a position where your muscle tone and posture are very poor. But as long as you understand and adhere to the principles and techniques, keep a steady rhythm, and follow the instructions to the letter, the rewards will be great—you will look and feel fantastic, and be brimming with a new vitality and confidence. Just remember to think tortoise, not hare!

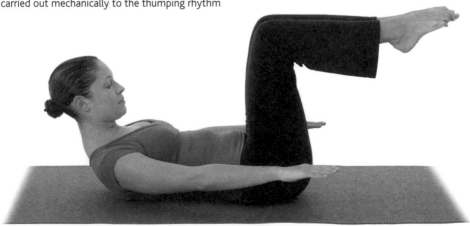

How to use this chapter

It is essential that you understand the principles of Pilates before you start practicing the movements, so it is suggested that you read through the whole chapter at least once, and then go back and familiarize yourself thoroughly with the techniques explained in the Body and Mind section. Work through the exercises in this section to help you master these techniques. You will then be ready to move on to the Warm-Ups and Introductory Level Exercises. It is suggested that you practice at that level at least twice a week for about six to eight weeks, working to gain stability of the central core and control of the deep abdominal and postural muscles. Once you feel confident, go on to the Beginner Level Exercises, again keeping stability in mind. When you are very familiar with the techniques, you can progress to the ultimate challenge: the Advanced Pilates moves. Some of the exercises are basically the same, with just a little extra challenge as you move up a level to help you progress; if you are unsure of a move, go back to the previous level until you feel ready to move on. Although Pilates is a very safe and gentle form of exercise, it is strongly advised that you take the precaution of obtaining medical clearance from your doctor before you start.

Step-by-step spreads

Introduction
This section outlines the aim of the exercise and the areas it benefits, and includes useful tips, advice and information.

Instructions
The step-by-step instructions are a clear, detailed guide to achieving the sequence of movements.

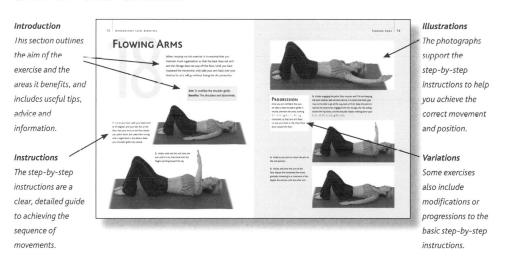

Illustrations
The photographs support the step-by-step instructions to help you achieve the correct movement and position.

Variations
Some exercises also include modifications or progressions to the basic step-by-step instructions.

THE HISTORY OF PILATES

Joseph H. Pilates was born in Düsseldorf in Germany in 1880. As a young child he suffered from a number of debilitating ailments, including asthma and rickets, which at that time would normally have left him severely crippled, if not permanently bedridden. But Pilates was blessed with a very positive attitude and, although he was so young, he was determined not to let his physical disabilities take over his life.

He began to study various methods of exercise and bodybuilding, but instead of concentrating on just one or two of these, he took the elements he required from all of them and developed his own method—which he later called "Contrology"—with great success. By his early teens, Pilates had grown into a fit and healthy individual, and he went on to become an enthusiastic sportsman, excelling in skiing, diving, gymnastics, and boxing. He could even include circus performer among his extraordinary list of achievements! Then, at the age of 32, he moved to England, where he became a professional boxer and taught self-defense to detectives at the police headquarters at Scotland Yard.

When World War I broke out two years later, Pilates was interned by the British authorities as a German national. He made constructive use of his time to develop his interest in creating and maintaining an optimum state of health, and the Pilates system was born of the belief that true well-being is achieved through a combination of physical fitness and a positive mental attitude. He shared his beliefs with his fellow internees, who were said to have remained exceptionally healthy as a result. He also set many seriously injured internees on the road to rehabilitation, helping them regain muscle tone by attaching springs to their beds to provide resistance as they carried out gentle exercise movements.

After the war, Pilates returned to Germany for a few years, where he worked with other pioneers of the movement technique. In 1926 he set sail for New York, and on the way met his future wife, Clara, who shared his radical views on health and fitness. The couple set up an exercise studio together, and soon met with growing success among people from a variety of disciplines. Pilates' method appealed particularly to dancers, actors, athletes, and gymnasts, who were keen to gain strength, vitality, stamina, and grace, but not the bulky muscles that went hand-in-hand with some bodybuilding techniques. What Pilates taught them was a holistic approach to health—his philosophy embraced total commitment to regular practice of the exercises, a diet that promoted physical and mental fitness, and that all-important attitude of determination and motivation. Pilates also helped clients suffering from injuries to a speedy recovery by making an immediate start on their rehabilitation. He designed a piece of equipment based on the experiments he had carried out with injured internees during the war: a sliding bed with springs that could be adjusted to suit the patient's stage of recovery. Equipment based on this concept is still used today in many modern Pilates studios.

Pilates may have started life as a weak, frail, sickly individual, but against all odds he recovered and remained healthy until his death at the age of 87, a shining example of the effectiveness of his approach to fitness. He wrote several books on the subject, including *Your Health* (published 1934) and *Return to Life Through Contrology* (1945). Nothing escaped his notice in his quest for optimum health—it is not by chance that several of the movements are reminiscent of a cat stretching. The "true" Pilates method was never formally taught or documented, and indeed, Pilates himself varied his method of teaching the exercises to meet the individual needs of his clients. This means that over the years practitioners have developed their own variations and methods of teaching the system— but they are all based on Pilates' excellent and enduring principles.

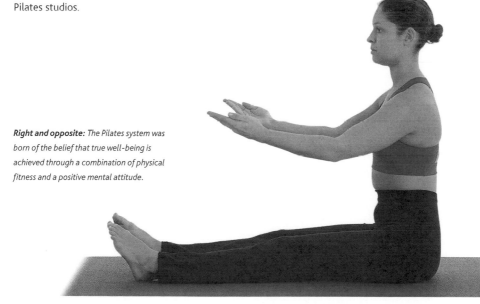

Right and opposite: The Pilates system was born of the belief that true well-being is achieved through a combination of physical fitness and a positive mental attitude.

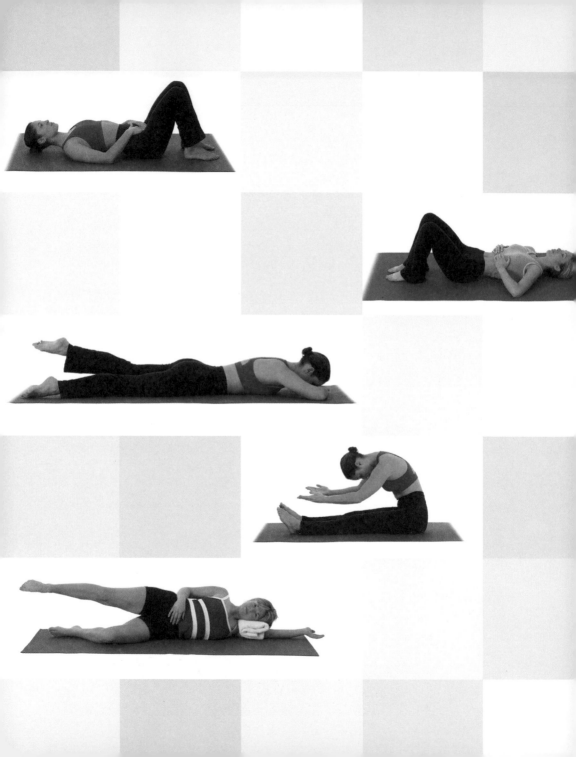

BODY AND MIND

VITAL TECHNIQUES

"We live in a modern society that loves shortcut techniques. Yet, quality of life cannot be achieved by taking the right shortcut. There is no shortcut, but there is a path. The path is based on principles revered throughout history. If there is one message to glean from this wisdom, it is that a meaningful life is not a matter of speed or efficiency. It's much more a matter of what you do and why you do it, than how fast you get it done."
Stephen R. Covey, *First Things*

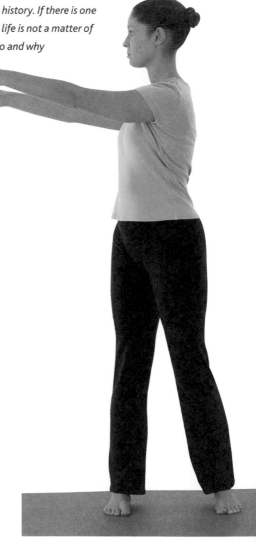

When Stephen Covey wrote this passage, he was talking about the organization and management of time—but his principles are appropriate to many things in life, including practice of the Pilates system. Pilates is a path toward a healthy body that functions at maximum efficiency. If you follow the path at the prescribed speed, adhering to the principles and techniques involved, you will get the result you want. If you try to stray from the path, hoping for a quicker result, you are likely to fail. So be patient, and learn to enjoy your steady progress. It may seem an impossible task at first, but it will be worth it!

There are many different exercises, ranging from warm-up exercises and beginners' exercises to advanced-level exercises; but the basic principles and techniques of Pilates are common to all levels, and are vital to the success of the exercises. To begin with, it is important that you take a little time to read through the following pages, and practice the exercises for breathing and abdominal hollowing— do not start practicing the Pilates movements, even at the warm-up level, until you are confident that you have mastered these basic techniques.

BREATHING

Breathing is something we do naturally and instinctively, without thinking, and we take it for granted that the way we breathe is the right way. Very often, however, our breathing is shallow, and we fail to take in sufficient air to oxygenate the blood properly. This in turn leaves us feeling tired and lethargic, adversely affecting both our energy levels and our spirits.

Controlled and effective breathing is vital to the Pilates technique, and mastering the art of breathing correctly is perhaps the steepest of the Pilates learning curves. Disciplines such as martial arts, t'ai chi, and yoga emphasize the importance of conscious breathing to help calm and focus the mind, release physical tension, and enhance learning —and Pilates is no exception.

To check if you breathe properly, lie down on the floor, breathe in through your nose and observe where that breath is going. If all that happens is that your upper chest moves a little, and then you exhale, your breathing is not effective. If you take a deep breath, pulling in your stomach tightly, then exhale and let everything go, your breathing is still not effective—in either of these cases, you will need to reeducate yourself.

The Pilates breath is wide and full into your back and sides, filling the lungs like bellows, expanding the diaphragm and pushing your ribcage out to the sides—imagine a bucket handle being lifted out. When you exhale, the diaphragm contracts, pushing all the stale air out of the lungs. Each step in the Pilates exercises begins with an instruction to inhale or exhale, and the movement accompanies the breath. You must have proper control over your breathing, so that the breath comes and goes in a steady, rhythmic, flowing way—otherwise, you will very likely find yourself holding your breath as you rush through the movement before collapsing in a breathless heap!

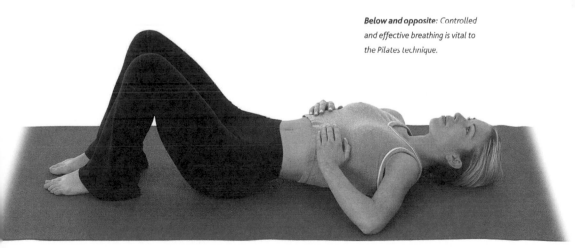

Below and opposite: *Controlled and effective breathing is vital to the Pilates technique.*

CENTERING

All movement comes from a strong, central "core"—the area below the base of the ribcage and above the line across the hip bones. Here, the transversus abdominis and the lumbar multifidus muscles together form an invisible "girdle of strength" around the body, which Pilates referred to as the "powerhouse." If you have poor posture or a bad back, this is an indication that your center is weak. The first aim of Pilates exercises is to strengthen this area by conditioning and toning the muscles to promote easy, flowing movement and good posture.

CONTROL AND CONCENTRATION

Mental and physical fitness is the result of a constant exchange of information and feedback between mind and body. While you are training, be focused on what you are doing—still your mind and allow it to listen to your body, and be aware of all sensations. Concentrate fully on each move so that you bring mind and body together to create a pattern of balanced and controlled movements, each one flowing slowly, gently, and gracefully into the next.

PRECISION

"The benefits of Pilates depend solely on your performing the exercises exactly according to the instructions." J.H. Pilates

Don't be tempted to do your own thing. Read the instructions carefully for each movement, and make sure you understand them before practicing the move. Carry out each move with precision; focus your attention on the relevant area of the body, make sure you are breathing fully and deeply, and inhale and exhale at the correct point in the exercise. Rushing through each movement and increasing the number of repetitions will not make it more effective—in Pilates, quality is far more important than quantity.

Left and opposite: Before you start practicing the Pilates technique, have a clear picture in your mind of what you want to achieve.

RELAXATION AND ALIGNMENT

Before starting your Pilates session, take a few minutes to relax your mind and body. It's important that your body is correctly aligned to enable you to carry out the movements in a natural, flowing way with ease and precision. Before you start any movement—whether you are standing, sitting, or lying face up or down—make sure:

- Your head is in alignment with your body and not tilted to one side or the other.
- Your shoulders are in line with your hips— imagine that your shoulder blades are sliding or "melting" down your back.
- Your knees are in line with your hips.
- Your feet are in line with your knees.
- Your back (see page 174) and pelvis (see page 175) are in "neutral."

MOTIVATION AND VISUALIZATION

Adopting and maintaining a positive mental attitude are key elements in the success of any new venture—without his positive outlook, Pilates would not have achieved his goal. It is a daunting prospect to make changes in your life, even though you know they will be of benefit to you, and it's all too easy to give up before you even start. Phrases such as "I can't do that" or "It's too late to change now" are unhelpful—so just don't use them! Instead, say firmly to yourself: "Yes, I can do that and I will succeed." Say it every day! You may feel silly at first, but you'll really appreciate it when the results of your efforts start to become visible to you. Before you start practicing Pilates, have a clear picture in your mind of what you want to achieve. It may be that you simply want to look and feel your best—long, lean, graceful, and brimming with self-confidence—or you may have physical problems that you wish to overcome, such as a bad back. Either way, Pilates is there to help you—provided you let it.

ANATOMY—BONES

One of the main aims of Pilates is to bring the skeletal system back to its natural alignment. The key points of the skeleton that are involved are the spine, the shoulder girdle, and the pelvis, which are all essential to maintaining good posture. Pilates also mobilizes the joints, and can help increase bone density, reducing the risk of osteoporosis and its associated problems, such as fractures.

THE SPINE

The spine is made up of 34 separate bones, called vertebrae. These form a column to protect the delicate spinal cord, a key part of the nervous system that delivers messages throughout the body from the brain, and returns messages from the body to the brain. The spine also connects and supports the rest of the skeleton.

Viewed from behind, the spine appears to be straight from top to bottom, but in profile you will see that it has four natural curves, which act as shock absorbers during movement. A number of the Pilates exercises instruct you to ensure that your spine is in "neutral." This means that you allow your spine to rest in its natural curves. If you are standing up, you should neither stretch out the spine unnaturally, nor slump so that the curves are exaggerated. When you are lying down, do not press your back into the floor or arch it so that the lower back comes up off the floor. Simply relax, so that your spine falls into its natural, neutral position.

When doing Pilates, you are also often asked to roll or unroll the back, one vertebra at a time. The vertebrae are joined together by ligaments, and cartilage disks between each vertebra prevent friction. This segmented, protected structure enables you to roll and unroll in a controlled, flowing way.

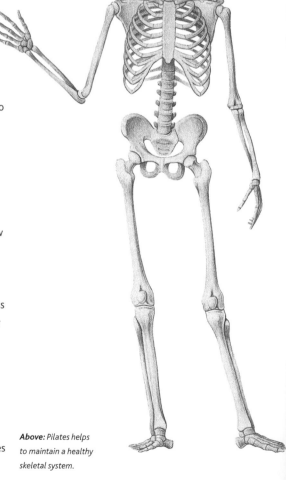

Above: Pilates helps to maintain a healthy skeletal system.

THE SHOULDER GIRDLE

The arms are joined to the torso at the shoulders. Three bones are attached to each shoulder: the clavicle, or collarbone, which is also joined to the top of the breastbone; the scapula, or shoulder blade; and the humerus, or upper arm bone. There is plenty of scope for bad posture stemming from the shoulders. We are often told to "stand up straight," but this may encourage you to pull your shoulders too far back into an unnatural position, causing strain across the collarbone and upper ribcage. You may habitually sit slumped forward, perhaps because your desk and chair are the wrong height, causing strain across the back, or your shoulders may have become unbalanced as a result of carrying heavy shopping. Tension is often carried in the shoulders, causing them to hunch up toward your ears. Finding the correct position for your shoulders is essential to creating good posture and correcting back pain.

THE PELVIS

The pelvis is joined to the lower part of the spine, and the legs are attached to the pelvis at the hip joints. A misaligned pelvis is another common problem, which can be caused by an unbalanced sitting position, for example, or by holding a baby propped on a hip. The abdominal muscles, which form part of the central "core," are attached to the pelvis at the pubic bone. Putting the pelvis into "neutral" means neither pushing it back (so that your bottom sticks out and your lower spine curves unnaturally), nor pushing it forward (so that your stomach sticks out and your spine is straightened). Again, the pelvis should be allowed to fall into its natural, neutral position so that it doesn't cause strain elsewhere.

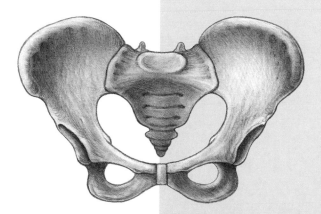

Above: A correctly aligned pelvis is essential to maintaining good posture.

ANATOMY—MUSCLES

Muscles are tissues that work together in pairs to create movement—as one muscle contracts, the other relaxes. To help you visualize this in action, hold out your arm in front of you with your hand palm-down and fingers pointing forward, parallel to the floor. Now let your hand flop down at the wrist—you can see how the muscles on the upper side of the wrist relax and stretch to allow the muscles on the underside of the wrist to contract. The more you pull your fingers back toward the underside of your wrist, the more the upper muscles have to stretch and the tighter the lower muscles become to allow the movement to take place.

Muscles need to be used regularly to keep them strong, and also stretched regularly to keep them flexible. Unfortunately, the modern inclination to travel everywhere by car instead of walking, coupled with the necessity to spend long hours sitting at a desk, means that many people do not give their muscles the attention they need to stay healthy. When muscles are not used very much, they become weak and lose elasticity, making movement more difficult—if you have ever had an illness that has kept you in bed even for just a few days, you will know how weak and wobbly you feel when you first get up and start to move again. Pilates recognized that prolonged lack of use, following

Above: Muscles need to be used regularly to keep them strong, and also stretched regularly to keep them flexible.

major illness or serious injury, led to the physical infirmity he suffered as a child, and he was a great believer in starting rehabilitation as early as possible to avoid unnecessary muscle wastage. (If you are recovering from a major illness or injury, always consult your doctor and a registered Pilates practitioner to advise you on a program of rehabilitation.)

Muscles are at their most powerful and effective when they are well toned but also relaxed. If your muscles have either become very tense (overcontracted) or are completely lacking in tone (overstretched), any movement can quickly lead to injury. An overcontracted muscle will stay tight even when you are not moving, and movement from an overcontracted muscle can lead to wear and tear on a joint as it tries to compensate by pulling toward the muscle. A weak, overstretched muscle can lead to instability around a joint, resulting in slow reflex actions. Pilates exercises aim to tone the muscles so that they are strong but flexible, enabling all movement to start from a state of relaxation.

The most important muscles targeted by the Pilates technique are those that form the "girdle of strength"—primarily the

Below: Strengthening the body's musculature to enhance support of the skeletal system is one of the main aims of Pilates, leading to greatly improved posture.

deep postural transversus abdominis and lumbar multifidus, supported by the pelvic floor muscles. If your abdominal muscles are very weak, you will need to devote some time to strengthening them, or you may find other, stronger muscle groups trying to take over the work. It is very tempting, for example, to engage the gluteus maximus—the buttocks—instead of the pelvic floor muscles, especially as you are more likely to be able to feel the contraction, or to try to flex the upper body by lifting the head and shoulders and tensing the muscles in the upper back. Once the abdominal muscles are strengthened and toned, however, all movement will become easier and more fluid, and you can then concentrate on working on muscle groups elsewhere, confident that you are supported by a strong center.

POSTURE

"Good posture can be successfully acquired only when the entire mechanism of the body is under perfect control."
J.H. Pilates

People with good posture look taller, sleeker, and more graceful than those who slouch. Good posture automatically makes you feel more confident, too.

On a physical level, we expect a lot from our bodies. We spend hours sitting at desks or driving; we wedge the phone between ear and shoulder so that we can work as we talk; we carry heavy bags, often favoring one side of the body. Poor posture can contribute to many ailments. The most obvious is back pain—you will be far less prone to this if you don't put unnecessary strain on the muscles through sloppy posture. But have you ever made the connection between poor posture and shortness of breath or irritable bowel syndrome? Correct posture allows your internal organs to work at optimum levels—for example, breathing will be more efficient if your lung capacity isn't restricted by your ribcage, and you are less likely to suffer from digestive problems if your stomach and intestines are not compressed.

Stand in front of a full-length mirror and look at yourself. Your shoulders should be level, with an equal distance between your ears and shoulders—this shows you are not pulling your body out of balance by tilting your head left or right. Your hips should be level, and also your kneecaps—if your weight isn't evenly distributed, there will be an overburdened joint or muscle somewhere in your body.

Now stand sideways to the mirror. Your head should be centered over your body and your spine should be erect but relaxed. Common postural problems include an exaggerated arch in the lower back, which throws the abdomen forward, or a slouch, which forces the head to fall forward, shortening the neck at the front and compressing the chest and abdomen.

Be honest! If you have inspected yourself in the mirror and you look good, but when you relax your posture collapses, you need to do some work. If you were cheating, your first instinct was probably to pull in your stomach, which automatically made you tuck in your tail, straighten your spine and head, and bring your shoulders into line with your ears. In other words, you pulled everything into correct alignment. When you strengthen the abdomen through Pilates, holding in your stomach will cease to be an effort, and even when you relax you will still retain good posture.

VISUALIZATION

To visualize something is to create a picture of the desired outcome in your mind's eye and to hold it there as a constant source of inspiration and motivation. If this sounds unrealistic to you, think about how often you visualize things without realizing. For instance, take a look around your living room, which is looking a little tired. You hate the wallpaper and would love to replace it with painted walls. Two new sofas would look great. The clutter needs sorting out and things you want to keep could be stored neatly instead. New curtains and fresh flowers instead of that dusty houseplant would complete the look. You see? You've created a clear image in your mind of a change you would like to make!

Try the same technique on yourself, and visualize a new you. Take a look at the jaded old you, with all your aches and pains and stresses reflected in your face and posture. Now visualize the new you: upright and confident, sleek and streamlined, glowing with health and vitality. Just hold the image in your mind, and focus on it as you are working with Pilates' technique. You can keep your goal in mind by hanging your favorite—but maybe a little too tight?—outfit where you can see it as you exercise, and visualize yourself fitting into it. Or try taking a photograph before you start, then take more at regular intervals so that you can see how well you have progressed —a visual source of motivation!

BIOFEEDBACK AND BODY AWARENESS

Biofeedback is a tool that will assist the mind-body connection. Most of us move around on automatic pilot, unaware of how it should feel to connect or contract a muscle correctly.

To raise your awareness of how one movement affects another part of the body, lie flat on the floor with your hands resting on your stomach in a triangle shape. The thumbs form the base of the triangle at the navel, and the fingers splay down to form a point at the pubic bone. Now imagine you have a glass of water balanced on the triangle and you are trying not to spill it. Focus your attention on drawing the navel back toward the spine in a gentle, controlled movement. You will feel the movement beneath your hands, but be conscious of what is happening to the pelvis and hips— unless they remain balanced and stable, that imaginary glass of water will spill!

When carrying out your Pilates exercises, keep that mind-body connection open all the time, giving and receiving constant feedback about the part of the body you are working on and how each movement affects the rest of the body.

Left and opposite: When you strengthen the abdomen through Pilates, holding in your stomach will cease to be an effort.

BREATHING

We have already seen that correct and effective breathing is essential to practicing Pilates—so take some time to learn the breathing technique. You are aiming for a gentle, non-exaggerated breath, and to breathe laterally, encouraging the ribcage to move out to the sides and back. The movement of the ribcage is described as "bucket handle"—as you inhale, the ribs move up and out, as if a bucket handle were being lifted, and as you exhale, the ribs move back to the center and slightly down, as if the bucket handle were being replaced. Go through the following exercise step by step, using your hands to give you feedback.

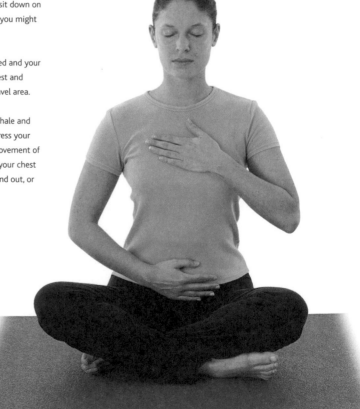

1. Find a warm, comfortable space and sit down on the floor. You will be here for a while, so you might like to sit on a cushion or a mat.

2. Sit upright, with your shoulders relaxed and your legs crossed. Place one hand on your chest and another on your stomach, around the navel area.

3. Close your eyes and for a moment inhale and exhale, as you would normally. Gently press your hands against your body, and feel the movement of your body as you breathe. You may feel your chest rise a little, and your stomach move in and out, or you may feel nothing at all.

NOTE

If you are breathing correctly, the chest and diaphragm should expand as you inhale, filling the lungs, and contract as you exhale, pushing the air out of the body.

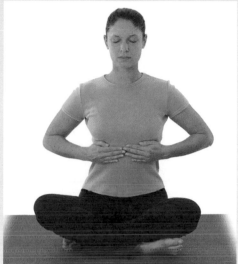

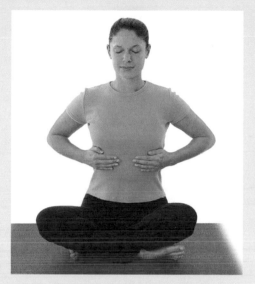

4. Now change your hand position. Close together the fingers and thumbs of both hands, as if you were going to make a chopping movement. Place the heel of each hand on either side of the ribcage, with the fingers extended to the soft opening at the center. Relax your shoulders and let the shoulder blades melt down your back.

5. Making sure there is no tension in the body, inhale through the nose and exhale with a sigh through a relaxed open jaw: remember the "H" sound in "hollow." Breathe in an even rhythm —try inhaling to a mental count of four and exhaling to a mental count of four. Maintain the relaxed position of your shoulders.

6. Now close your eyes, and sense within your body how you are feeling. You should be sitting comfortably, with your hands on the ribcage, shoulders relaxed, and the breathing flowing to a gentle rhythm.

7. With the heels of your hands, apply gentle pressure to the ribcage—make your mind and body aware of the area. Inhale gently as if breathing in to the heels of your hands, feeling your ribcage expand to the sides; as you exhale, feel the ribs closing into the center. Repeat for nine more breaths. Get a sense of the flow feel the "bucket handle" move out and up, in and down.

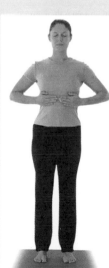

VARIATIONS

Try the same technique standing up, lying on your back or face down, or in the crook position (sitting up with your knees bent at 45 degrees, feet flat on the floor). It will be easier to find the connection in some positions than in others, but you should still try them all in preparation for carrying out the exercises.

BODY PLACEMENT AND MUSCLE SYNERGY

CORE CONDITIONING

Pilates is a synergistic activity: this means that for each individual movement in each exercise—whether you are working at the most basic or the most advanced level—every part of the body is working together to bring about the desired result. As we have already seen, the first priority with Pilates is to create the strong, stable "center" or "core"—which Pilates referred to as the dynamic "girdle of strength" or "powerhouse"—from which stems perfect posture as well as all movement.

When you are practicing the Pilates technique, you will frequently come across the instruction to "maintain the connection with the center," and until you can do this with complete ease and without effort, you will not be able to focus all your attention on the area you are working. So what is this all-important center, and where do you find it?

Well, loosely speaking, it is the area located between an imaginary line running around the body just below the diaphragm and another running above the pelvic floor. It is three muscles found within this area that are engaged to create a strong center. These are the muscles that stabilize the lower spine in the lumbar region of the back, and they are positioned very deep and close to the spine itself: the transversus abdominis to the front of the spine and the lumbar multifidus to the back, both in line with the navel, and the pelvic floor muscles at the base.

The transversus abdominis is one of the four muscles that make up the abdominal wall, and is the deepest of the four. To help you locate the position of this muscle, stand so that you are straight but relaxed, take both hands and grab your sides with your thumbs around your waist pointing toward your back, and your fingers pointing in toward the navel. When you have a firm hold, give a good cough! As you cough, you will feel a muscle bounce beneath your fingers. Now take a breath in, and then blow out—you will feel the same muscle bounce again. This is the transversus abdominis (TVA) and, because it is such a vital component in core stability, it is essential to learn how to engage it properly.

TVA ACTIVATION

As with everything, there is a right way and a wrong
way to go about activating the TVA. Let's start
with the wrong way, which is simply to overdo it
by sucking in your abdomen with such gusto that
it's almost sticking to your spine. What you are
aiming for is to master a gentle contraction of the
TVA—one that you can maintain easily at all times,
whether you are standing still, walking, exercising,
or sitting, and either working at a desk or relaxing in
your favorite comfortable chair.

To understand the reason for this, you need
to know that there are two types of muscles –
mobilizers (task muscles) and stabilizers (postural
muscles). Muscles that mobilize are responsible for
large movements, such as kicking or throwing—they
mobilize the limbs. Compared to stabilizers, they
are superficial (closer to the surface), longer, work
harder (at approximately 40–100 percent of their
power) and are "phasic"—that is, they tire quickly,
so they work in phases for short periods, turning on
and off.

Muscles that stabilize are close to the spine or
lie deeply; they are shorter than mobilizers, work
for longer periods, and are tonic (that is, they hold
tone). Stabilizers need endurance and so they work
at only about 20–30 percent of their maximum
voluntary contraction (MVC). The TVA is a stabilizer
muscle—a deep, postural muscle—so this is why it
is important to work it gently.

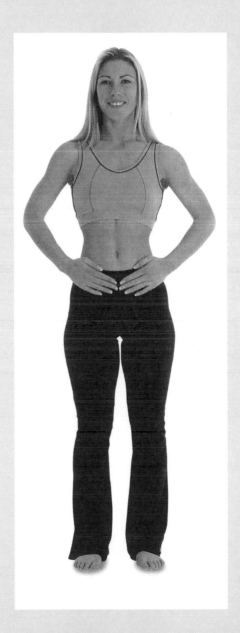

*Right and opposite: Before practicing the Pilates technique,
you must learn how to locate and correctly activate the
transversus abdominis muscle (TVA).*

WORKING THE **TVA**

How do you recognize when you are working at the correct level of TVA contraction—30 per cent? Read this exercise through, then try it out.

Stand up, keeping good posture in mind—stand tall, with your knees slightly bent, but not locked, your tailbone pointing toward the floor, and your shoulders relaxed, as though your shoulder blades were melting down your back toward your pelvis. Hold your head upright, so that your ears point toward the ceiling, and focus your eyes on the horizon. In this position, you will feel elongated—stretched from head to toe. Now let your stomach relax as far as it will go—and give this position a score of 0 percent. Return to the first position.

Now pull everything in so that your whole body feels sucked in and tense—pull your stomach into your spine and elevate your shoulders until they are almost touching your ears. You should now bear a strong resemblance to Frankenstein's monster! Give this position a score of 100 percent, so the yardstick is 0 percent for no tone and 100 percent for tense to the point of being unable to breath.

To get to 30 percent, return to the first position again, standing tall but relaxed. Take your right hand and place your thumb at the lower edge of your navel, then splay your fingers and span your hand until the little finger is toward the pubic bone, resting your hand on your stomach. Draw your navel in and up toward your spine, away from your hand, to 100 percent, then release it halfway to 50 percent while retaining your

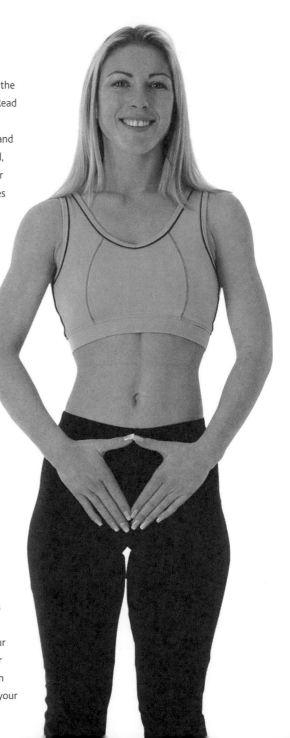

elongated stance—do not slump. Now release a little farther, and you have reached 30 percent—you should have a sensation of feeling connected but not tense, in a position that you can maintain all day and every day, whatever you are doing.

ENGAGING THE PELVIC FLOOR

The pelvic floor muscles are an important element in stabilizing the spine, working in conjunction with the TVA. A gentle contraction is sufficient to activate the pelvic floor—do not be tempted to clench the buttocks in an effort to feel the tension. Lie on your back and place your hand on the lower abdominal area, then gently exhale, and draw up the muscles from below and in front of the pelvic area—as you do so, you will feel the TVA contracting.

NEUTRAL PELVIS

The pelvis is the basis of support for the body—your spine rests upon it and your legs move from it, so for optimum movement the pelvis should be "organized" in the best possible postural position. This position is described as "neutral."

To help you identify the perfect position, lie on your back with your knees bent to 45 degrees, your feet flat on the floor, and your body relaxed. Place your hands in a triangle over your stomach, with your thumbs forming the base of the triangle at the navel, and your fingers splaying toward the pubic bone to form the point. When the pelvis is properly organized, your palms should be flat on your lower stomach muscles, and your hip bones should be positioned evenly on either side of your hands. If your fingers are raised higher than your thumbs, your pelvis is in a posterior tilt, and if your thumbs are higher than your fingers, it is because your pelvis is in an anterior tilt. When your pelvis is in neutral, your hands will be absolutely level, with your spine neither too flat to the floor nor arched to the ceiling. The "Neutral to Imprinted Spine 50/50" exercise on page 220 helps you to settle into this position.

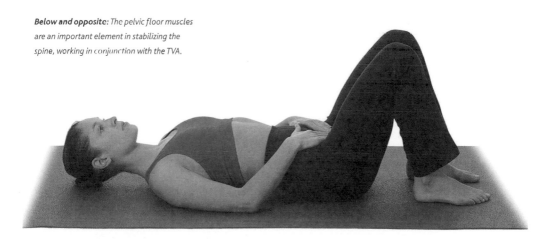

Below and opposite: The pelvic floor muscles are an important element in stabilizing the spine, working in conjunction with the TVA.

ABDOMINAL HOLLOWING

Abdominal hollowing is created when the deep postural abdominal muscles are contracted, and is the result of correct breathing. As we have already seen, it is essential to inhale and exhale gently, and not try to force the breath. As you inhale, you should get a sense of the ribs moving to the sides and the back, not up and away. As you exhale, drawing the navel in and up toward the spine, you should get a sense of the ribs closing in and moving toward the hips as if on railroad tracks. If you force the breath out, you will engage the external oblique muscles and end up with a bulging, dome-shaped abdomen —not what you want at all! Practice with the following exercise.

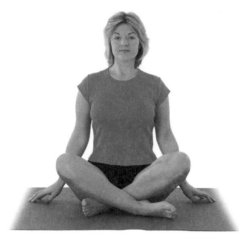

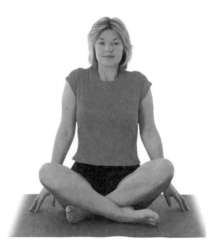

1. Stand or sit comfortably and elongate the spine, lengthening through the crown of your head to the ceiling, and through your tailbone to the floor.

2. Shrug your shoulders to your ears, then roll gently backward, letting your shoulder blades glide down your back toward your pelvis.

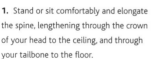

3. With your shoulders relaxed, place one hand on either side of your ribcage, with your fingertips facing each other at the opening between the ribcage. Inhale gently, and feel your ribcage moving gently out toward the sides.

4. Exhale gently, relaxing the jaw and sighing softly through an open mouth. Draw up on the pelvic floor and back on the navel toward the spine to a maximum of 30 percent, as described earlier (see page 184), feeling the ribs move in toward the center and gently downward, creating the hollow—a "slope" from the ribs to the pelvis. If you exhale to the "H" sound of "hollow," it will open the mouth and drop the jaw, helping you resist the temptation to either blow out or force the exhale through pursed lips.

LENGTHENING THE NECK

All Pilates movements are geared toward realigning the body into a perfect posture, with the spine in optimum alignment. The neck—the top of the spine, or "cervical spine"—is a very important part of this process. Maintaining correct alignment in the neck is particularly important when you are flexing the upper body off the floor. It's tempting to lift with the shoulders and head, jamming the chin into the chest or, even worse, hanging the head backward like a hinged lid.

To lengthen the neck in preparation for flexing the upper body correctly from a strong central core, rock the chin SLIGHTLY toward the chest, without lifting your head—you should feel as if someone has taken your head in both hands and gently stretched it away from your shoulders. Your neck will now remain in alignment.

Right: Directing your gaze at the horizon when you are carrying out the Pilates movements will help the movement flow as well as helping you maintain alignment.

THE GAZE

When you walk along gazing at the floor, your head is downcast and your posture slumped forward—but look up and focus your gaze on the horizon, and you will stand tall and upright, with your head and neck in alignment with your spine. Perfect!

Directing your gaze at the horizon when you are carrying out the Pilates movements will help the movement flow as well as helping you maintain alignment. If you are doing a sit-up, for example, and you keep your gaze on the ceiling, your head will fall back, compressing your neck and spine. If you allow your gaze to follow the horizon as you move, however, so that it is focused in front of you at knee level when you reach the top of the movement, your head and neck will be aligned and in the optimum position. This is a good example of the synergistic nature of Pilates—you will find it progressively easier to direct your gaze correctly as your center becomes stronger and more stable. Your center will become stronger when you allow it to do its work and do not inadvertently substitute other muscle groups by directing your gaze incorrectly.

BEFORE YOU START

ENVIRONMENT

It is essential to find a quiet, comfortable place for your Pilates session, where you will not be disturbed. If you can allocate some time when you are alone at home, this is ideal—turn off the telephone, ignore the doorbell, and focus all your attention on yourself. If there are usually other family members at home when you are, be firm about claiming some time for yourself—it's easier to do this if you can schedule in a regular time. Make sure the room you work in is warm but well ventilated, and that you have plenty of space to lie down with your arms outstretched.

You will not need any special equipment, but working on a padded exercise rug or a folded blanket is essential to protect your spine from bruising. A full-length mirror is also useful, so that you can keep a constant check on your position—what you think you are doing and what you are actually doing may not be the same!

CLOTHING

Choose light, comfortable clothing that allows you to move without restriction—fairly close-fitting leggings or cycling shorts with a T-shirt or leotard top are ideal as they are totally flexible and will move with you. It's best to exercise in your bare feet, but you can wear socks if you prefer.

WHEN TO EXERCISE ...

Pilates exercise can be done at any time, and there are advantages to both ends of the day. Pilates can be energizing in the morning, especially if you normally find it difficult to come alive early in the day, while in the evening it is useful for unwinding. The best time to exercise is really a matter of personal preference and knowing when you are most likely to be able to enjoy quiet time for yourself.

If you choose the morning, make sure you warm up sufficiently before you start, because your muscles will not have had a chance to get mobilized, and ensure that you have enough time to focus on what you are doing— you will not be able to concentrate fully otherwise.

... AND WHEN NOT TO EXERCISE

Do not exercise if you are feeling at all unwell, or have not fully recovered from a recent illness. You must also avoid exercise after eating a heavy meal or drinking alcohol, or if you are taking painkillers—whether over-the-counter or prescribed—because these will mask any warning signs of injury.

It is important that you are neither cold nor stressed when you start exercising. Deep breathing for a few minutes is an excellent way to destress—find a quiet, comfortable place to do this, and imagine that you are releasing your stresses as you exhale, and taking in peace as you inhale.

Walking on the spot for a few minutes, or taking a short, brisk walk outside in good weather will help release both mental and physical tensions. It will also warm you up at the same time by getting your circulation going—if you start exercising when your joints and muscles are chilled, you are far more likely to injure yourself. Don't be tempted to warm yourself up by taking a hot bath, as this will relax your muscles rather than boost your circulation.

PRECAUTIONS

Although Pilates is a perfectly safe form of exercise for everyone, at any age, there are still some things you should consider. As with any exercise program, it is important to consult your doctor before you start if you are receiving treatment for a medical condition, have not exercised regularly for some time, if you have had a significant injury, or if you are pregnant, postmenopausal, or suffer severe menstrual symptoms.

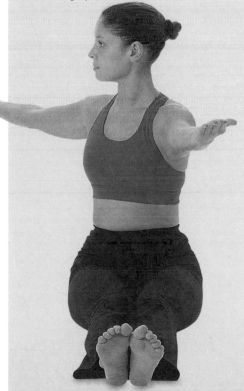

Right and opposite: *Choose light, comfortable clothing and go barefoot to allow unrestricted movement when you are carrying out the Pilates exercises.*

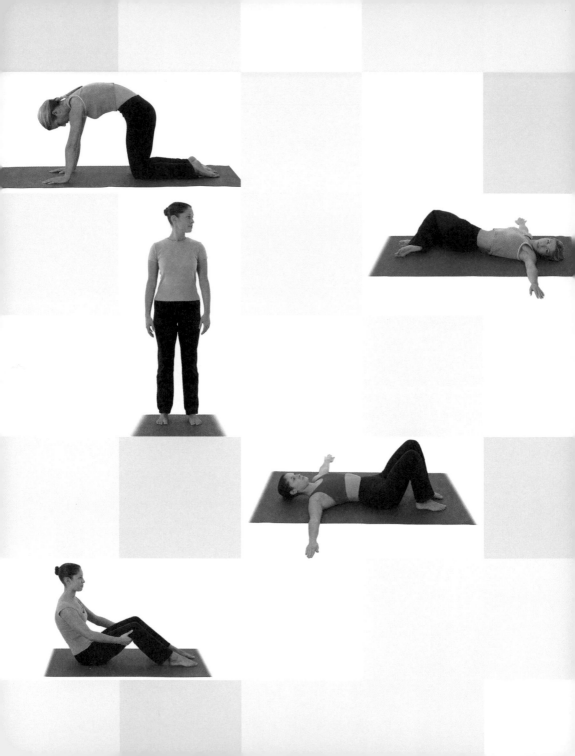

WARM-UPS

INTRODUCTION

The warm-up exercises on the following pages will help you release any tension held in the mind or body before you start on your Pilates session. They will also mobilize and stabilize the central core and stretch all the muscles in preparation for the more demanding exercises. It is essential to do these warm-ups, whether you will then be moving on to the Introductory, Beginner, or Advanced Level exercises.

If you are completely new to the Pilates system, you can limit your session to the warm-up exercises only, just for a week or two, while you start to put into practice the techniques and principles you learned in the previous section. The gentle actions will make you aware of the importance of developing the really strong, stable central core from which all movement stems. They will get you used to relaxing the shoulder girdle, spine, and pelvis into the neutral position, engaging the pelvic floor and abdominal muscles, and breathing laterally as you carry out the exercises, as well as inhaling and exhaling at the appropriate moment.

At first, repeat each movement only three to five times (on each side of the body, where relevant), carefully observing your body's reaction to the moves. As you become familiar with the warm-up, increase the number of repetitions—adding an extra one at each session – to a maximum of ten. Relax,

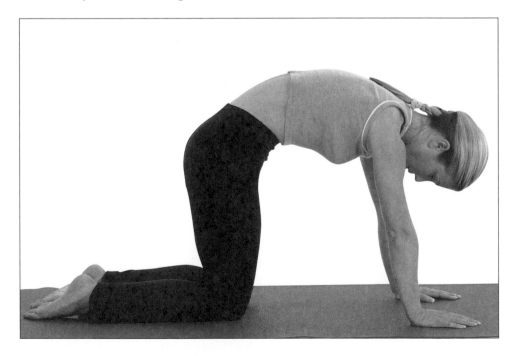

concentrate, and work slowly and steadily, following the instructions precisely. Do not try to push any of the moves too far, too soon—you are making progress the whole time, even if it does not seem that way. Always keep the principles in mind and always think "quality."

It is also a good idea to keep just to the warm-up movements for a short while if you have not taken any form of exercise for some time and perhaps feel stiff and inflexible as a result. You may find that this stage is enough of a challenge in itself at first, but in no time at all you will have loosened up your joints and started to improve your muscle tone, and you will feel ready, able, and keen to tackle the next step.

The warm-up exercises are also ideal for mobilizing you first thing in the morning—after all, no self-respecting cat would wake up after a long sleep and start moving about without first having a good stretch in all directions! And they are a quick

and effective way to iron out the kinks—both in the body and the mind—that tend to accumulate during a busy working day. Remember, however, that the warm-up exercises are not a "quick fix"—you must always put the full amount of focus and concentration into preparation and execution.

Most importantly, do remember—at whatever stage you are at—to think positively and keep visualizing your goal as you work through each movement. There's that fit, healthy, and confident new you out there, either waiting to be discovered or anxious to be maintained!

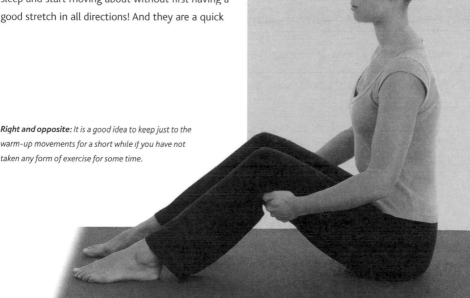

Right and opposite: It is a good idea to keep just to the warm-up movements for a short while if you have not taken any form of exercise for some time.

FOCUS ON BREATH

Aim: To focus your attention on your posture and breathing.

Benefits: The mind and the whole body.

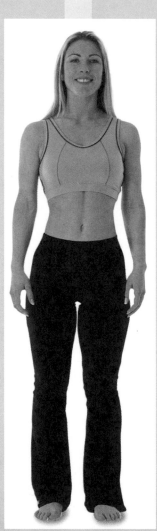

1. Stand upright, with your shoulders and spine in neutral. Place your feet hip-width apart, keep your knees soft, and let your arms hang loosely by your sides.

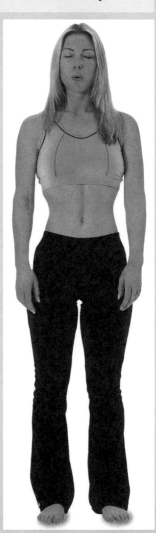

2. Close your eyes and focus on your breathing. Inhale through your nose, and visualize clean, energizing air entering your body and filling your lungs.

SHRUGS

Aim: To release tension from the neck and shoulders.
Benefits: Shoulders, neck, and upper body.

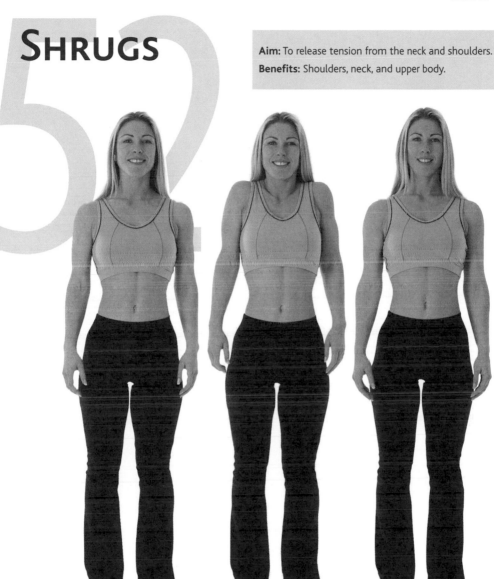

1. Stand upright with your shoulder girdle and spine in neutral. Place your feet hip-width apart, keep your knees soft, and let your arms hang loosely by your sides. Focus on your breathing, with eyes closed if you wish.

2. Inhale, and lift your shoulders up toward your ears.

3. Exhale, and draw the shoulder blades into neutral. At first, do the shrugs five times, increasing to a maximum of ten.

ROLLING DOWN

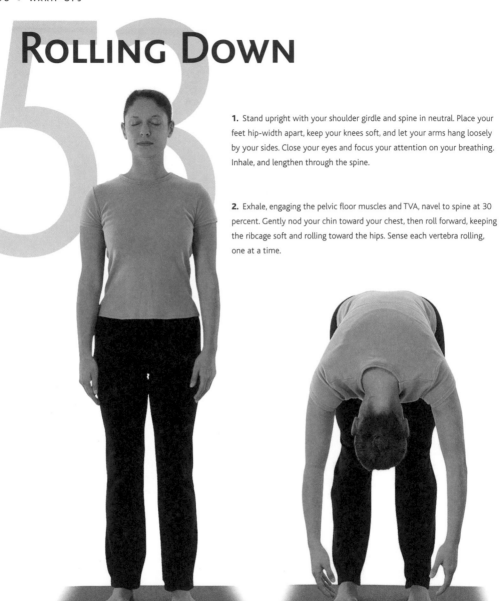

1. Stand upright with your shoulder girdle and spine in neutral. Place your feet hip-width apart, keep your knees soft, and let your arms hang loosely by your sides. Close your eyes and focus your attention on your breathing. Inhale, and lengthen through the spine.

2. Exhale, engaging the pelvic floor muscles and TVA, navel to spine at 30 percent. Gently nod your chin toward your chest, then roll forward, keeping the ribcage soft and rolling toward the hips. Sense each vertebra rolling, one at a time.

Aim: To mobilize the spine and connect with the center.

Benefits: The spine, shoulders, and upper body.

3. Only roll down to your point of comfort—do not try to go too far too soon. At the bottom of the move, inhale, feeling the air inflate your spine and keeping the pelvic floor muscles and abdominals engaged.

4. Roll back up, one vertebra at a time. As you finish the roll, exhale and release the shoulder blades to neutral. At first, do the roll five times, increasing to a maximum of ten.

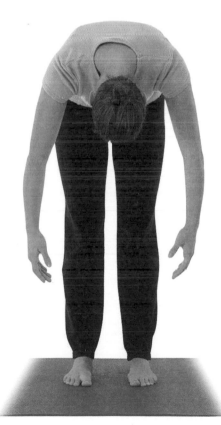

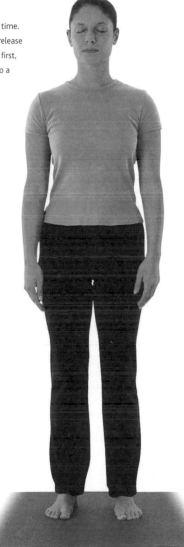

HEAD TURNS

54

Aim: To release tension from the neck.
Benefits: The neck and shoulders.

1. Stand upright with your shoulder girdle and spine in neutral. Place your feet hip-width apart, keep your knees soft, and let your arms hang loosely by your sides. Inhale, to prepare.

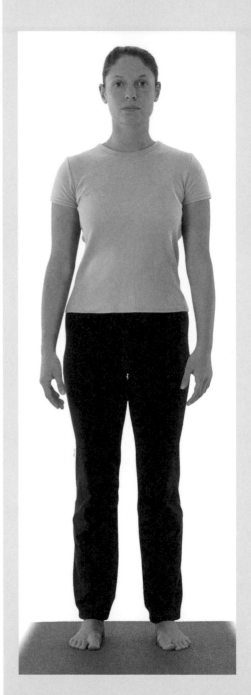

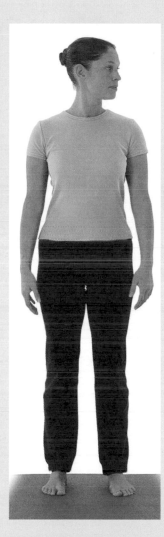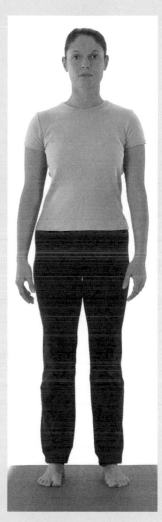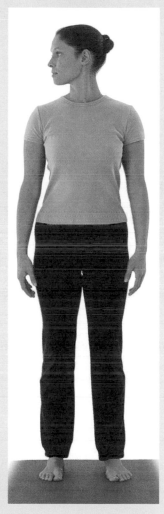

2. Exhale, engaging the pelvic floor muscles and TVA, navel to spine at 30 percent. Turn your head to look over your left shoulder, keeping your head in line with your gaze on the horizon.

3. Inhale, and return to center. Repeat the movement five times in this direction.

4. Repeat the movement five times in the opposite direction.

PIVOT

Aim: To mobilize the whole body and promote coordination.

Benefits: The spine, shoulders, hips, arms, and legs.

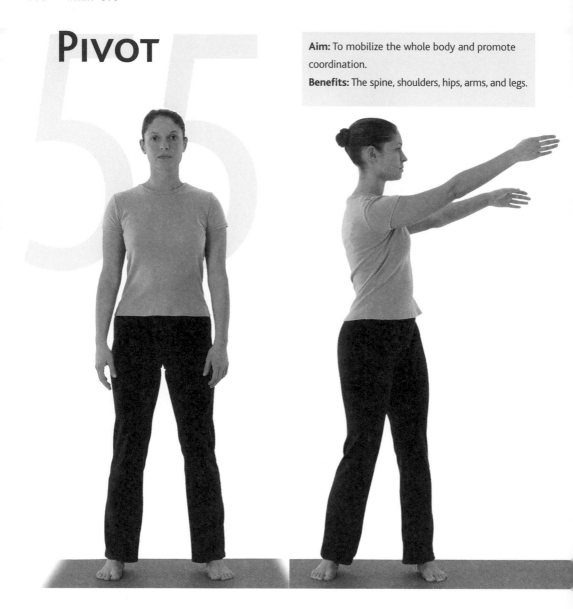

1. Stand upright with your shoulder girdle and spine in neutral. Place your feet wider than hip-width apart, keep your knees soft, and let your arms hang loosely by your sides. Inhale, engaging the pelvic floor muscles and TVA, navel to spine at 30 percent. Lengthen through the spine.

2. Exhale, and twist your body to one side. Let your arms swing loosely, moving with you. Your legs will also twist with the movement.

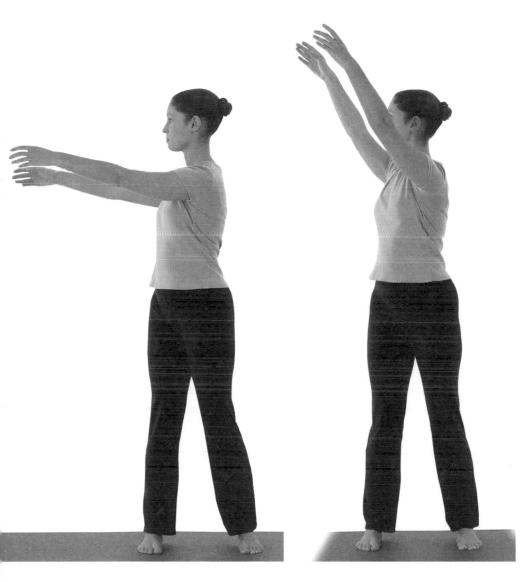

3. Inhale, and twist back to the center. Exhale, and twist to the other side. Inhale, and twist back to the center.

4. Each time you twist, raise your arms higher, until they reach over your head, then work them back down to your sides, in a continuous, flowing movement. Take three twists in each direction to get to the top of the movement, and three more twists in each direction to get back down.

SHELL STRETCH

56

Aim: To stretch and lengthen the spine.

Benefits: The spine, shoulders, neck, and abdomen.

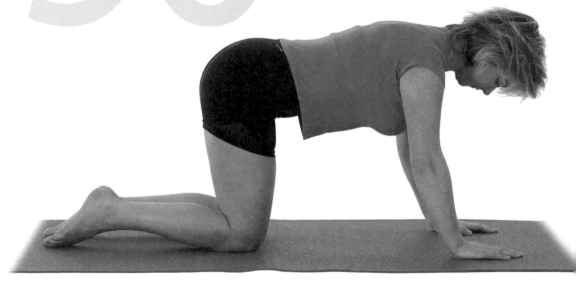

1. Kneel on all fours, with your knees under your hips and your arms in line with your shoulders, with the elbows soft but not locked. Drop your head between your arms. Inhale, to prepare.

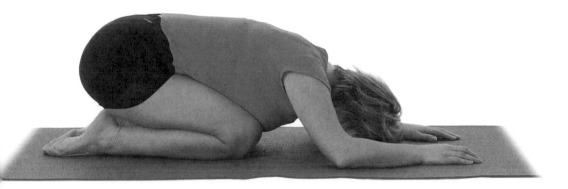

2. Exhale, engaging the pelvic floor muscles and TVA, navel to spine at 30 percent. Lower your bottom to your heels, keeping your hands on the floor in front of you and your head resting between your elbows. Hold this position for 15–20 seconds as you inhale and exhale, keeping the center connected. Feel the spine lengthen on the inhale.

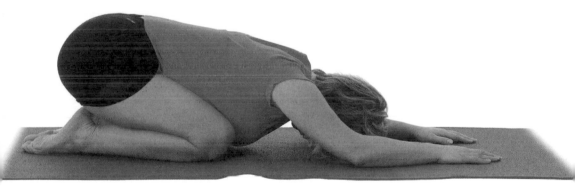

3. Inhale, and lift your bottom off your heels. Move your hands out 3–4 in (8–10 cm) farther, then exhale and lower your bottom back to your heels, keeping the center connected. Again, hold this position for 15–20 seconds as you inhale and exhale, keeping the center connected. Feel the stretch in the upper back and shoulders on the inhale. Exhale, and relax.

PROGRESSION

Once you are at ease with this movement, you can increase the intensity of the stretch.

Starting from Step 2, ease your buttocks off your heels and "walk" your hands a further 6–8 in (15–20 cm). With both palms down flat and your head between your elbows, ease your buttocks back toward your heels. This time the stretch will also be felt in your upper back and shoulders.

CAT STRETCH I

57

Aim: To mobilize the spine and help with stabilization.
Benefits: The spine, shoulders, neck, and abdomen.

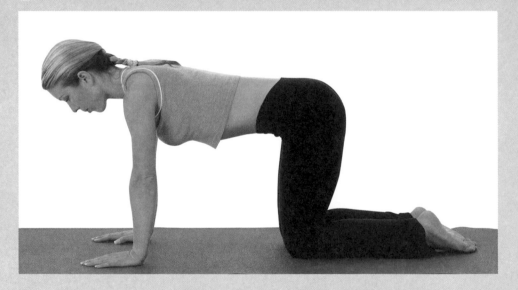

1. Kneel on all fours, with your spine and shoulder girdle in neutral, your knees under your hips and your hands under your shoulders. Keep your elbows slightly bent, but not locked. Inhale, keeping your body in neutral.

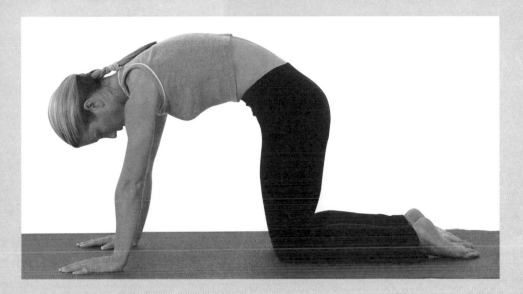

2. Exhale, engaging the pelvic floor and pulling your navel back to your spine. Keep the abdominals scooped to the spine for support. Flex the spine, curling from the tailbone toward the head. Inhale at the top of the movement.

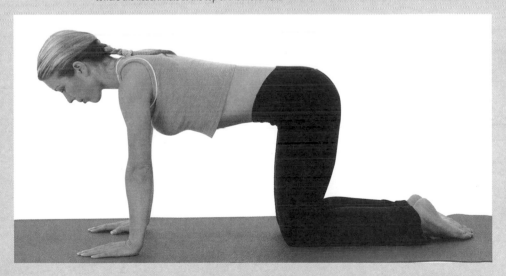

3. Exhale, and lengthen through the spine to the start position, keeping the spine in neutral. Inhale, to prepare. Exhale, and repeat the movement. Start with five repetitions and increase to a maximum of ten.

MERMAID (SIDE BEND)

58

Aim: To stretch and flex the spine, with the core connected.
Benefits: The shoulders, neck, spine, and abdominals.

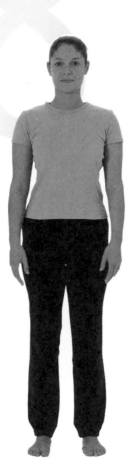

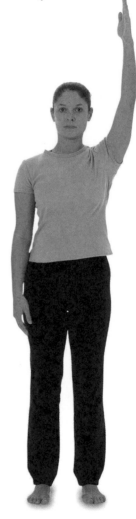

1. Stand upright with your shoulder girdle and spine in neutral. Place your feet hip-width apart, keep your knees soft, and let your arms hang loosely by your sides.

2. Standing tall and relaxed, inhale and take the left arm above your head, with the fingers pointing toward the sky. Stretch through your fingers, keeping the arm strong.

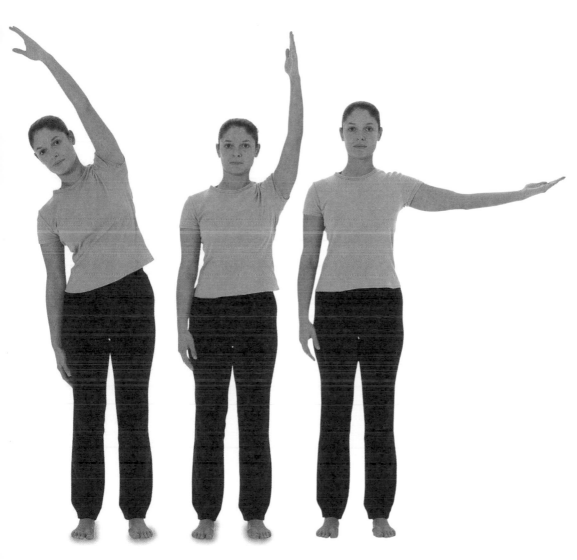

3. Exhale, and side bend to the right, keeping your pelvis in neutral. Allow your head and arm to follow your spine.

4. Inhale, and float back up to center, keeping your arm extended.

5. Exhale, and let your arm flow back down by your side. Slide your shoulder blades back into neutral, making sure there is no tension in the head, neck, and shoulder complex. Repeat the movement to the left. Do a total of five side bends on each side.

C-CURVE 1

59

Aim: To mobilize the spine and strengthen the central core.
Benefits: The spine, neck, shoulders, and abdominals.

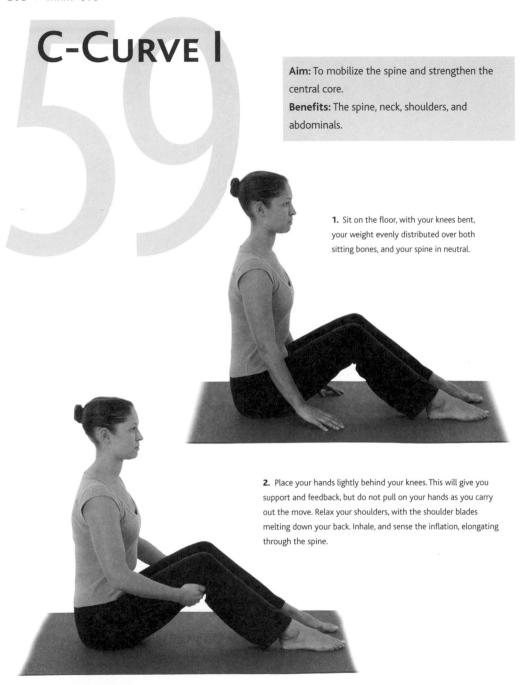

1. Sit on the floor, with your knees bent, your weight evenly distributed over both sitting bones, and your spine in neutral.

2. Place your hands lightly behind your knees. This will give you support and feedback, but do not pull on your hands as you carry out the move. Relax your shoulders, with the shoulder blades melting down your back. Inhale, and sense the inflation, elongating through the spine.

3. Exhale, engaging the pelvic floor muscles and TVA, navel to spine at 30 percent. Rock back off the pelvis toward the floor.

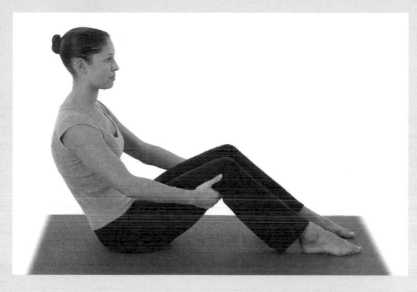

4. Pause, inhale, and return to the upright start position. Keep the abdominals scooped and hollowed throughout the whole move for support. Only go as far as you can each time without shuddering or lifting your feet off the floor. Repeat the movement five times, increasing to a maximum of ten.

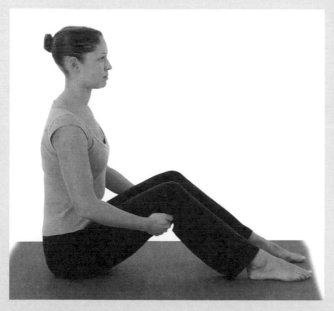

MODIFICATION

Relax your feet and lift your toes, resting only your heels on the floor. This will take the tension out of your hip flexors and so release the muscles.

TRUNK ROTATION

Aim: To strengthen and stabilize the central core.
Benefits: The neck, abdomen, and hips.

1. Lie on your back, with your knees bent and your feet flat on the floor. Extend your arms to the sides of your body at shoulder level, with your palms down. Relax your spine and shoulder girdle into neutral, and allow your chest to soften. Engage the abdominal and pelvic floor muscles.

2. Inhale, wide and full.

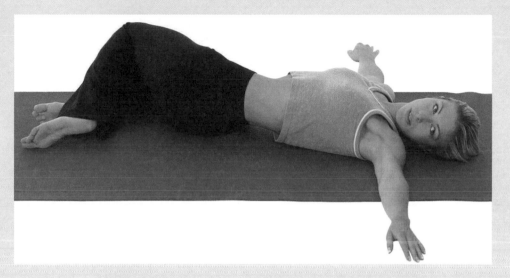

3. Exhale, and roll your knees to the right, keeping your head in neutral and both shoulders connected to the floor, with the shoulder blades in neutral. Inhale.

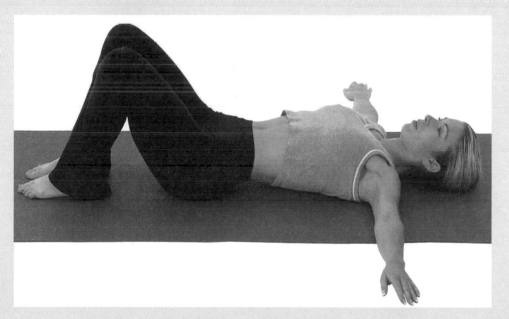

4. Exhale, as you return your knees to the center. Repeat the movement in the opposite direction. Do the exercise a total of five times in each direction.

SHOULDER SHRUGS

6

Aim: To release any tension created in the shoulders during the warm-up.
Benefits: The shoulders, neck, and spine.

1. Lie on your back, with your knees bent and your feet flat on the floor. Extend your arms to the sides of your body at shoulder level, with your palms down. Allow your chest to soften.

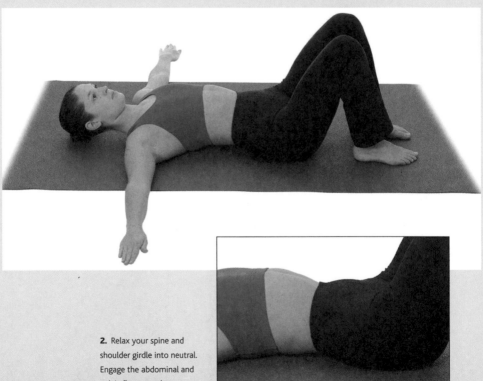

2. Relax your spine and shoulder girdle into neutral. Engage the abdominal and pelvic floor muscles.

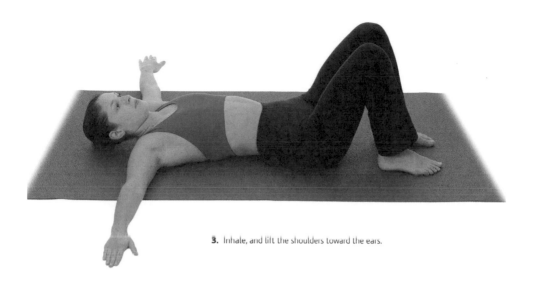

3. Inhale, and lift the shoulders toward the ears.

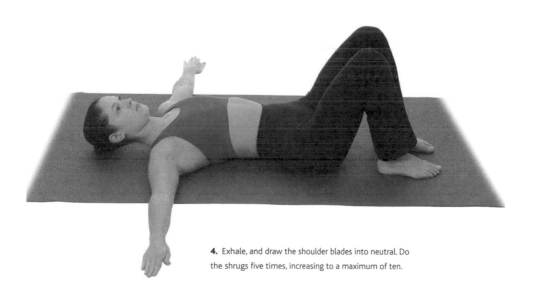

4. Exhale, and draw the shoulder blades into neutral. Do the shrugs five times, increasing to a maximum of ten.

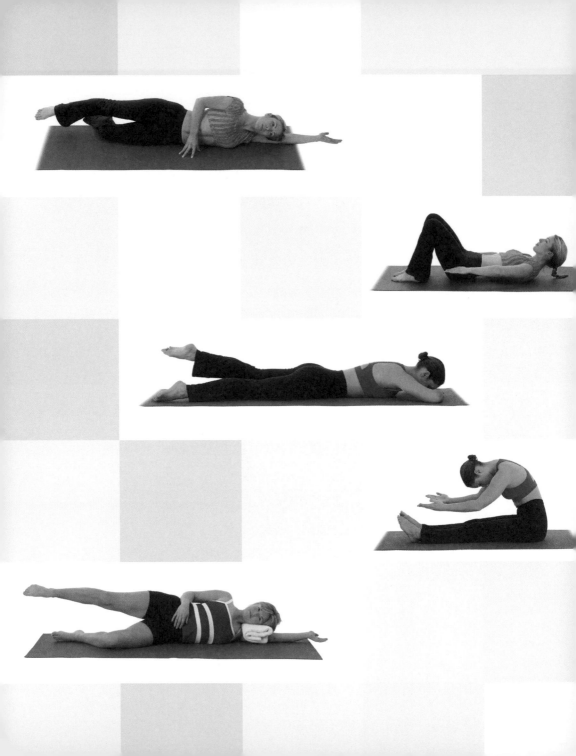

INTRODUCTORY LEVEL
EXERCISES

INTRODUCTION

When you arrive at the stage where you are ready to start practicing the introductory level exercises, do the warm-up exercises followed by these exercises at least twice a week for about six to eight weeks. At first, repeat each movement only three to five times, building up to a maximum of ten times. Remember to work on each side of the body, where relevant, and as always, aim for slow and steady progress.

Some of the movements in this section will already be familiar to you from the warm-up section, and will reinforce the process of strengthening and stabilizing the central core. Read each exercise carefully and make sure you understand it before you start working through the steps. Take it gently, making sure you inhale and exhale at the right points, and that you keep the center connected—it's easy to let these things go while you are concentrating on the intricacies of the move itself. Remember the importance of precision!

This section introduces the Pilates leg exercises. They are very effective, and as long as you pay attention to detail, you will get fantastic results in the hip and thigh areas. Detail in this case means aligning the body correctly by keeping the pelvis in neutral and the hips stacked one above the other. It also means working the muscle in the optimum position. Do not simply swing the leg up and down or raise and lower it aimlessly—make sure you really experience the movement, feeling the muscle as it lifts and lowers your leg. Have total control over both the up phase and the down phase—it will help to imagine that you are working against some form of resistance, such as gently flowing water.

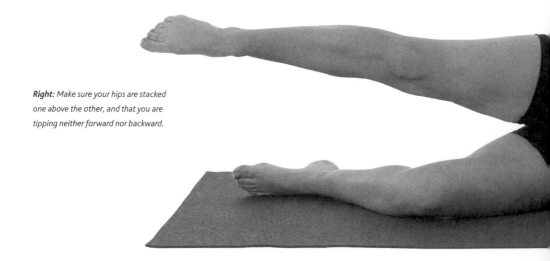

Right: Make sure your hips are stacked one above the other, and that you are tipping neither forward nor backward.

Follow these simple guidelines to help you achieve and maintain the correct alignment when you are lying on your side for the leg exercises:

- Make sure your hips are stacked one above the other, and that you are tipping neither forward nor backward—place your upper hand across your navel with your fingertips on the floor to give you some support and feedback.
- Position the bottom leg in a figure 4 to give you a stable base (as you advance, you narrow the angle, making the base of support less stable, until eventually the angle is only very slight).
- When you have one arm extended away from you and your leg or legs extended to a point at the toes, make sure you are positioned in a straight line through the head and body from fingertip to toe, with no grip or tension in the shoulder.
- Keep the body steady, without movement except in the working leg.
- Keep the top shoulder relaxed, with the shoulder blade gliding down toward your pelvis—the shoulder should not move throughout the exercise, so a glass of water could be safely placed there!
- When raising and lowering the leg, do not make huge movements—lift to an angle of about 30 degrees, and lower to hip height.
- Keep the center connected, with the pelvic floor drawn up and the navel drawn back toward the spine, and resist the temptation to let the stomach muscles contract and relax.

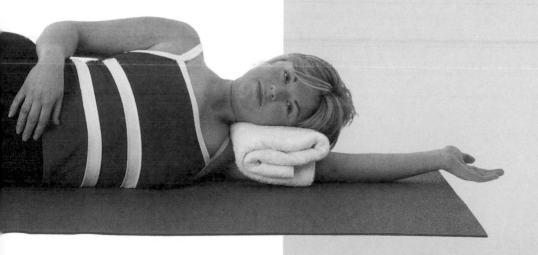

BREATHING

Aim: To strengthen the central core by activating the transversus abdominis through breathing.
Benefits: The transversus abdominis, lumbar multifidus, and pelvic floor muscles.

You will be lying on your back for many of the Pilates exercises. This exercise will help you learn to stay relaxed and connected with your breathing while you are in this position.

1. Lie on your back, with your knees at 45 degrees, your feet flat on the floor, hip-distance apart, and your shoulder girdle in neutral. Rest your hands palms down, one on either side of your ribcage.

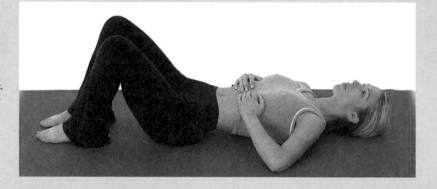

2. Inhale wide and full, feeling your ribcage expand and your breath going into your back and sides.

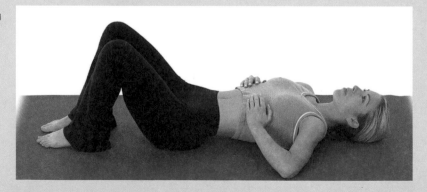

3. Exhale, gently drawing up the pelvic floor and activating the TVA in and up (MVC 30 percent). Feel your ribcage close in and soften, as if funneling down to the hips.

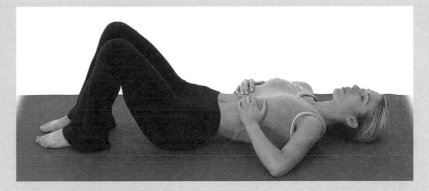

4. Continue to inhale and exhale as above, focusing your attention on your breathing. At first, inhale and exhale five times, increasing to a maximum of ten.

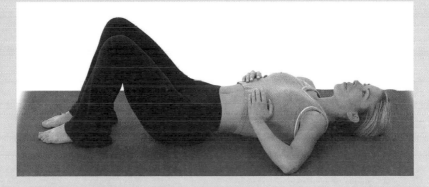

5. Remember your breathing is gentle, not forced. Exhale through the mouth, keeping the jaw relaxed, and do not be tempted to blow through pursed lips.

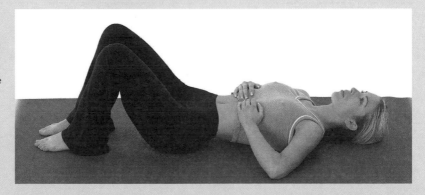

NEUTRAL TO IMPRINTED SPINE 50/50

Aim: The aim of this exercise is simply to help you position the spine in neutral when you are lying on your back.
Benefits: The pelvis and the spine.

1. Lie on your back, with your knees at 45 degrees and your feet flat on the floor. Place your hands on your stomach, making a triangle with your thumbs in a line at the base of your navel and your fingers splayed downward, coming together to make a point at the pubic bone (this will provide feedback as you carry out the movement). Relax your shoulder girdle and spine into neutral.

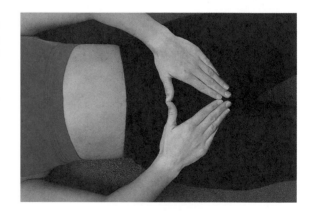

2. Inhale wide and full, feeling your ribcage expand and your breath going into your back and sides.

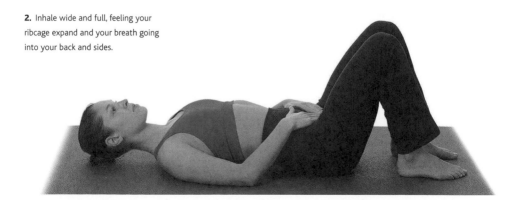

3. Exhale, engaging your pelvic floor muscles and TVA. Simultaneously, draw the pubic bone toward the navel and gently tilt the pelvis toward you, rolling your tailbone off the floor. You need to identify with the position of the lower abdominals at the front of the body, from the navel to the pubic bone, so imagine this movement as a "grab" from the front, rather than a push from behind.

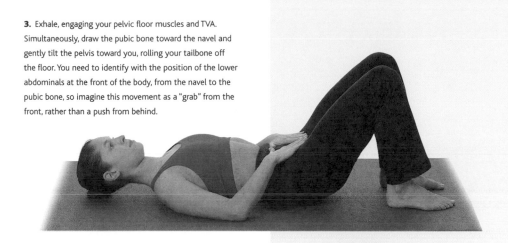

4. Inhale, and release the pelvis to neutral. Exhale, and arch the back gently.

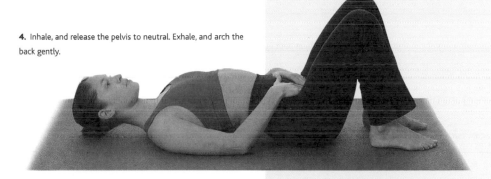

5. Inhale, and release the pelvis to neutral. Repeat the inhale and the exhale five times each at first, increasing to a maximum of ten. Check that the pelvis has come back to neutral properly each time.

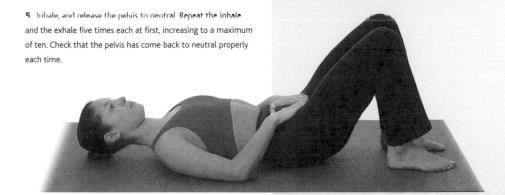

LOWER ABDOMINALS I

Aim: To strengthen the central core.
Benefits: The lower abdominal muscles.

This is a challenging exercise as you need to maintain the
core connection while breathing naturally. You also need to
make sure you are activating the tilt from the muscles of the
lower abdominals and not the gluteus maximus (buttocks).

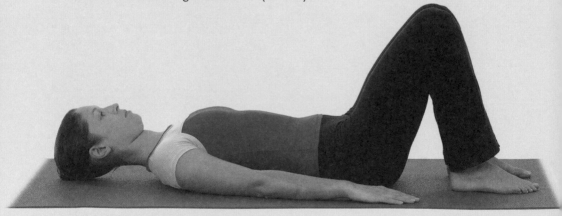

1. Lie on your back, with your knees at 45 degrees and your feet flat on the floor,
hip-distance apart. Either rest your arms at your sides, palms down, or lay your hands
in a triangle on your stomach as in the previous exercise (*see* page 220). Relax your
shoulder girdle and spine into neutral.

2. Inhale wide and full.

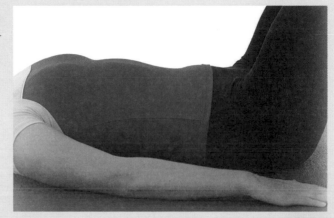

3. Exhale, draw up the pelvic floor muscles and draw back the navel to the spine to 30 percent. Simultaneously, draw the pubic bone toward the navel and, using your abdominals, gently tilt the pelvis toward you, rolling your tailbone off the floor. As in the previous exercise, this is a "grab" from the front, not a push from behind.

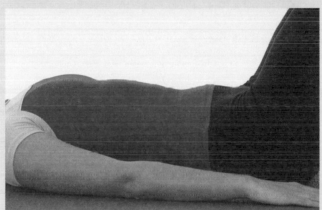

4. Inhale, and hold the tilt, keeping the TVA contraction activated at 30 percent. Exhale, as you roll back to neutral. Repeat the exercise five times at first, increasing to a maximum of ten. Each time, hold the position for one inhale and one exhale, keeping the abdominals scooped and hollowed. As you become familiar with the movement, you can progress to two inhales and two exhales as you hold the position, and then gradually increase to a maximum of ten inhales and ten exhales.

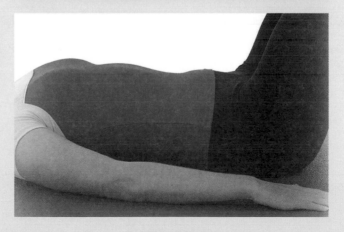

ABDOMINALS 1

Aim: To flex the spine and strengthen the central core.
Benefits: The neck, shoulders, spine, and abdominals.

1. Lie on your back, with your knees at 45 degrees and your feet in line with your knees. Rest your arms by your sides, palms down. Lengthen your neck, and relax your upper body, keeping your shoulder girdle neutral.

2. Inhale and lengthen through the back of your neck by gently nodding or rocking your chin to your chest. Do not jam your chin into your chest or raise your head—just imagine your neck lengthening on the floor.

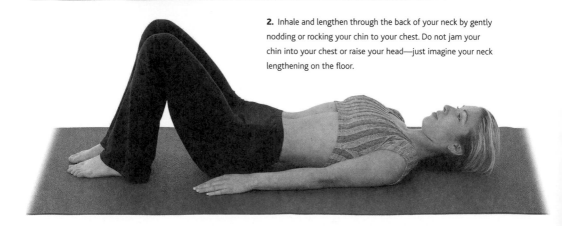

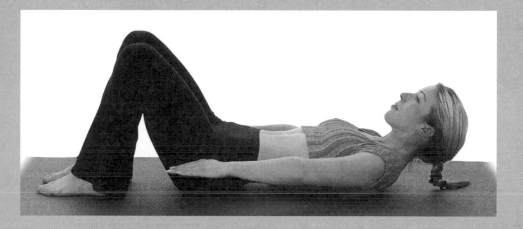

3. Exhale, activate the pelvic floor and navel to spine (30 percent), then flex forward, allowing your head and shoulders to curl off the floor and bringing your ribcage toward the pelvis. Raise your arms off the floor, level with your shoulders. Make sure your pelvic floor muscles and TVA are engaged, navel to spine, and that your spine remains neutral. Do not lead with the head and shoulders—let the flexion (muscle bending) come from the center. Inhale, maintaining flexion. Make sure the pelvic floor stays drawn up and you maintain navel to spine. Resist the temptation to release the body back—keep focused forward, with the abdominals hollowing out.

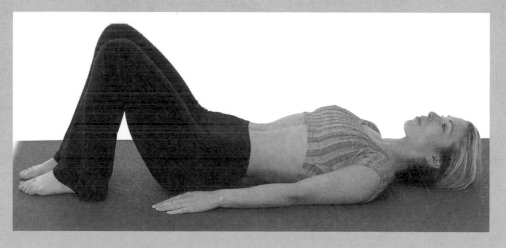

4. Exhale, and lower and roll the body back to the floor. Repeat the movement five times at first, increasing to a maximum of ten.

Leg Slide

66

Aim: To stabilize the pelvis.

Benefits: The center connection and the hip flexors/extensors.

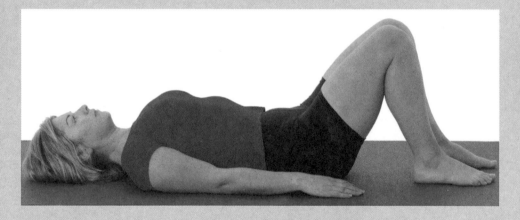

1. Lie on your back, with your knees bent at 45 degrees and your feet flat on the floor. Rest your arms by your sides, palms down and elbows slightly bent. Relax your shoulder girdle and spine into neutral and engage the pelvic floor and navel to spine. Inhale, wide and full.

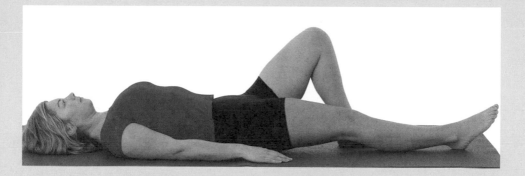

2. Exhale, drawing up and back, and slide one leg away along the floor until it is fully extended, keeping the heel in contact with the floor. Inhale, keeping your leg straight.

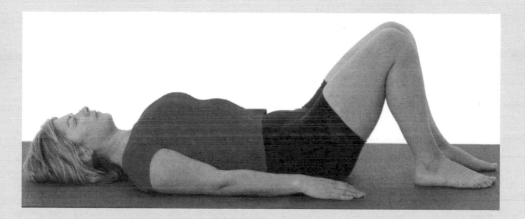

3. Exhale, draw up and back, and slide the leg back up to 45 degrees. Repeat the movement five times, then change to the other leg. Increase the repetition to a maximum of ten on each leg.

PROGRESSION

As you become familiar with this exercise and your stabilization improves, you can progress to alternating the legs. However, make sure that you are strong enough to do this without rocking the pelvis.

KNEE FOLDS

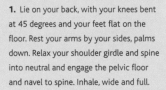

Aim: To stabilize the pelvis, strengthen the lower abdominals, and mobilize the hips.

Benefits: Transversus abdominis and hip flexors/extensors.

1. Lie on your back, with your knees bent at 45 degrees and your feet flat on the floor. Rest your arms by your sides, palms down. Relax your shoulder girdle and spine into neutral and engage the pelvic floor and navel to spine. Inhale, wide and full.

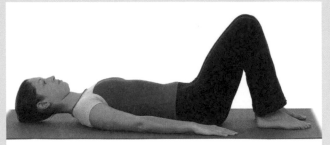

2. Exhale and allow one knee to float slowly up toward the ceiling, as if being pulled by an invisible string. Stop when the knee is in line with the hip and the angle of the knee is 90 degrees. Inhale, maintaining 30 percent TVA activation and keeping the leg bent at 90 degrees.

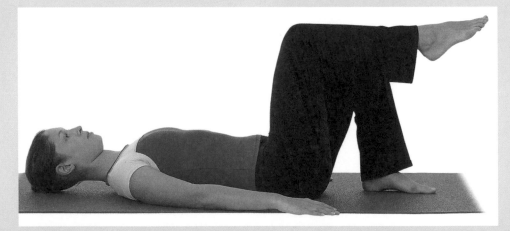

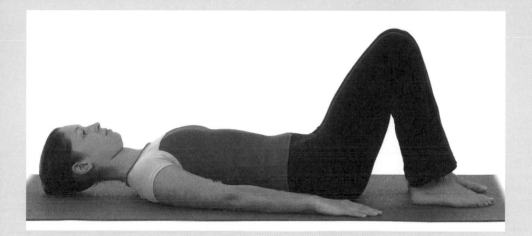

3. Exhale, lowering your foot to the mat with the knee bent at 45 degrees. Do not allow the back to arch as you return the foot to the floor, and keep the center connected and strong.

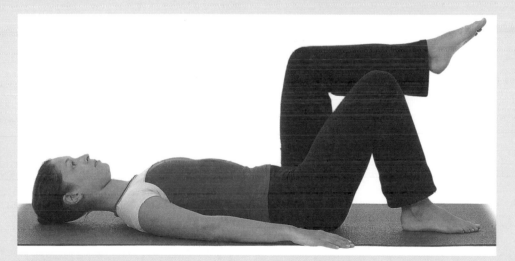

4. Repeat the movement five times, then change to the other leg. Increase the repetition to a maximum of ten on either leg.

PROGRESSION

As with the previous exercise (*see* page 226), you can progress to alternating the legs once your stabilization improves. Make sure that you are strong enough to do this without rocking the pelvis. Be very careful not to let the abdominals dome and the back arch as you replace the foot to the floor.

FLOWING ARMS

When carrying out this exercise, it is essential that you maintain trunk organization so that the back does not arch and the ribcage does not pop off the floor. Until you have mastered the movement, only take your arm back over your head as far as it will go without losing the rib connection.

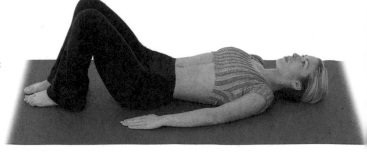

Aim: To stabilize the shoulder girdle.
Benefits: The shoulders and abdominals.

1. Lie on your back, with your knees bent at 45 degrees and your feet flat on the floor. Rest your arms on the floor beside you, palms down, but make them strong, with a slight bend in the elbows. Relax your shoulder girdle into neutral.

2. Inhale, wide and full, and raise one arm until it is at chest level with the fingers pointing toward the sky.

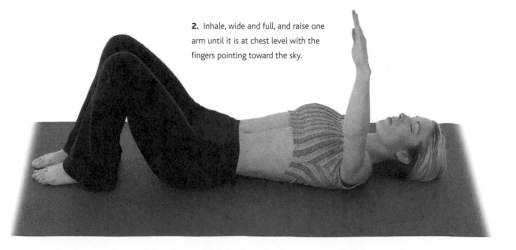

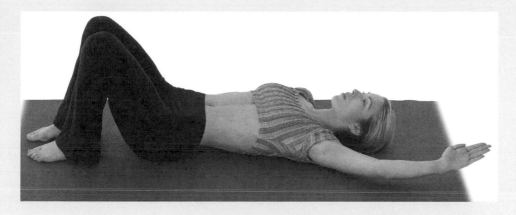

PROGRESSION

Once you are confident that you are able to keep the pelvic girdle in neutral, alternate the arms, working them both together in a flowing movement, so that one arm flows up over your head as the other flows down toward the floor.

3. Exhale, engaging the pelvic floor muscles and TVA and keeping the spine neutral. Take the arm back as if to touch the floor (you may not be able to go all the way back at first). Keep the pelvis in neutral, the abdominals engaged with the ribcage, the ribs sliding toward the hip bones, and the shoulder blades melting down your back, with the shoulder girdle stable.

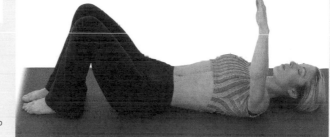

4. Inhale as you start to return the arm to the mid position.

5. Exhale, and lower the arm to the floor. Repeat the movement five times, gradually increasing to a maximum of ten. Repeat the exercise with the other arm.

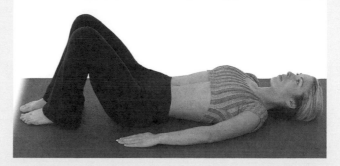

TRUNK ROTATION

In this exercise you rotate your head in the opposite direction to your legs, being careful to maintain the shoulder connection to the floor.

Aim: To strengthen and stabilize the central core.
Benefits: The neck, abdomen, and hips.

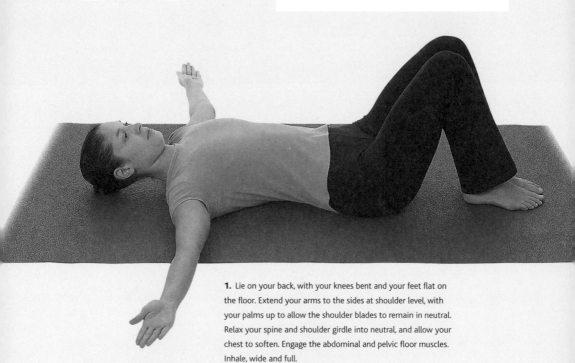

1. Lie on your back, with your knees bent and your feet flat on the floor. Extend your arms to the sides at shoulder level, with your palms up to allow the shoulder blades to remain in neutral. Relax your spine and shoulder girdle into neutral, and allow your chest to soften. Engage the abdominal and pelvic floor muscles. Inhale, wide and full.

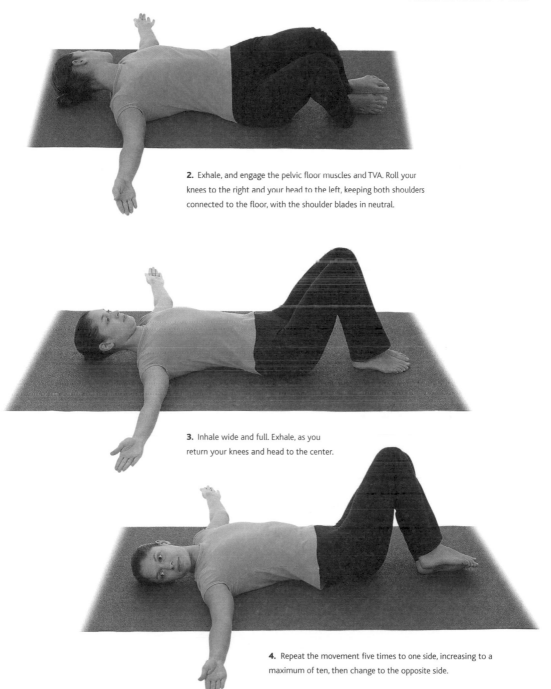

2. Exhale, and engage the pelvic floor muscles and TVA. Roll your knees to the right and your head to the left, keeping both shoulders connected to the floor, with the shoulder blades in neutral.

3. Inhale wide and full. Exhale, as you return your knees and head to the center.

4. Repeat the movement five times to one side, increasing to a maximum of ten, then change to the opposite side.

C-CURVE II

70

This is a progression of the warm-up exercise on pages 208–209. This time, position your hands lightly on the sides of your knees. Try to unroll farther each time you practice the movement but only go as far as you can comfortably without losing form.

Aim: To mobilize the spine and strengthen the central core.
Benefits: The spine, neck, shoulders, and abdominals.

1. Sit on the floor, with your weight evenly distributed over both sitting bones and your spine in neutral. Relax your shoulders, with the shoulder blades melting down your back. Inhale, and sense the inflation, elongating through the spine.

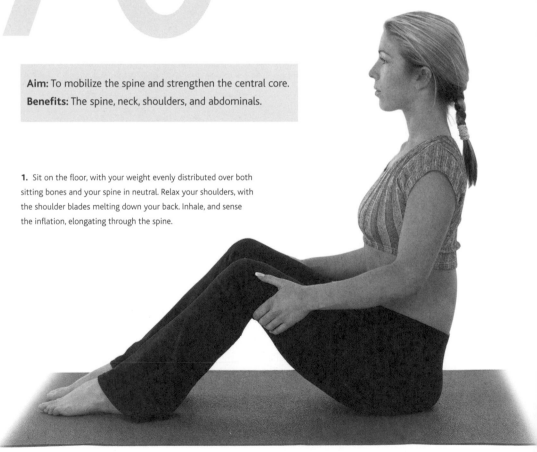

2. With the points of your toes gently touching the floor, engage the pelvic floor muscles and TVA navel to spine at 30 percent. Connect with the center, slowly roll backward off the pelvis. Rock slightly back and forth.

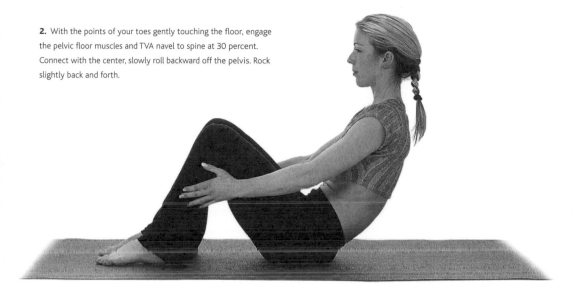

MODIFICATION

Relax your feet and lift your toes, resting only your heels on the floor (this will take the tension out of your hip flexors).

3. Balancing on your toes, inhale as you roll back to the start position. Repeat the movement five times, gradually increasing to a maximum of ten.

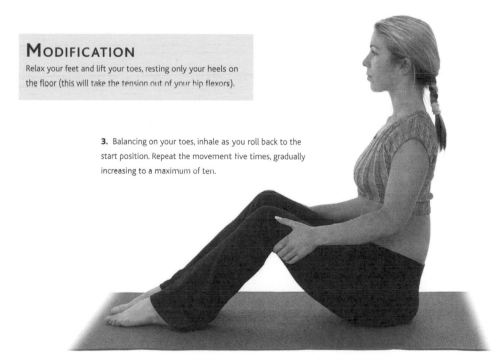

SWAN DIVE I

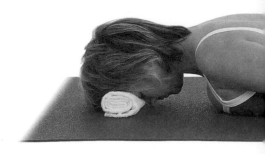

1. Lie face down, with your forehead resting on the floor on a folded towel or soft pillow. Rest your arms by your sides, palms down, and relax your shoulders into neutral. Keep your inner thighs connected and your toes pointed. Exhale, engaging the pelvic floor muscles and TVA.

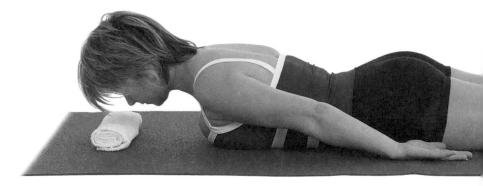

2. Inhale, peeling your upper body off the floor from the hips. Lengthen through the back, pulling your shoulder blades down. Keep the abdominals engaged for support. Keep the chest wide open and the shoulders in neutral. Keep your eyes focused on the floor and do not push back the neck and head.

3. Exhale, and lower your upper body to the floor, drawing in the navel and pelvic floor. Repeat the movement five times, increasing to a maximum of ten.

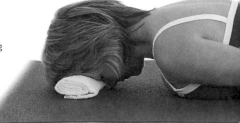

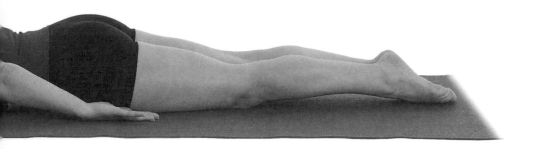

Aim: To strengthen and stabilize the shoulder girdle and spine, and work the spine extensors.

Benefits: The shoulders, spine, transversus abdominis, hamstrings, and gluteus maximus.

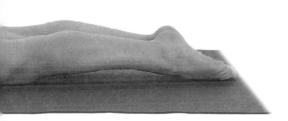

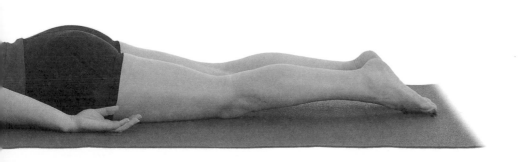

SPINE STRETCH I

Aim: To lengthen the muscles of the spine.
Benefits: The neck, shoulders, spine, hips, and abdominals.

1. Sit on the floor, with your weight evenly distributed over both sitting bones, and your legs extended hip-width apart (if the hamstrings are too tight, bend your knees slightly or sit on a rolled-up towel or mat). Lengthen your spine, so that the crown of the head is reaching toward the ceiling. Extend your arms in front of you, slightly below shoulder level, palms facing up. Relax the shoulder girdle into neutral. Inhale, and lengthen the spine, lifting up from the hips.

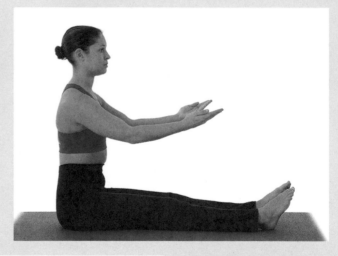

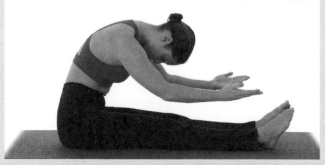

2. Exhale, engaging the pelvic floor and TVA. Curl the chin to the chest, but do not force it. Keep the abdominals scooped so that the ribs float to the hips. Curl out toward your feet as if rolling over a large beach ball.

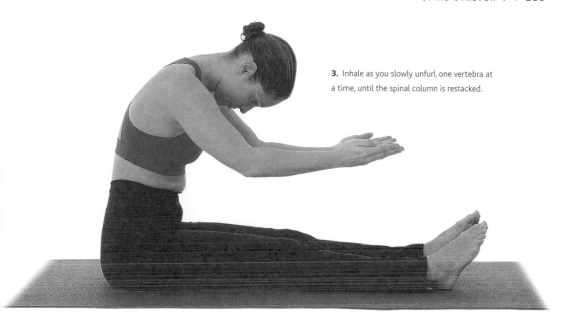

3. Inhale as you slowly unfurl, one vertebra at a time, until the spinal column is restacked.

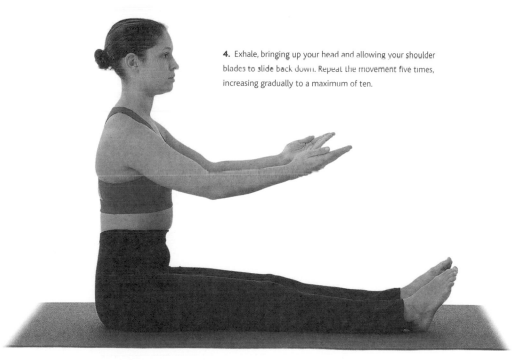

4. Exhale, bringing up your head and allowing your shoulder blades to slide back down. Repeat the movement five times, increasing gradually to a maximum of ten.

SWIMMING I

73

Aim: To lengthen the spine and legs.
Benefits: Shoulders, spine extensors, and transversus abdominis.

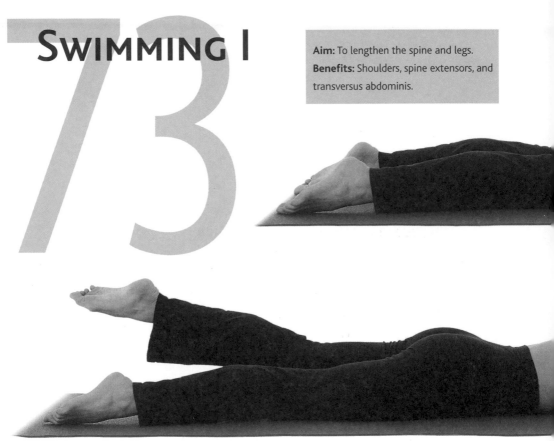

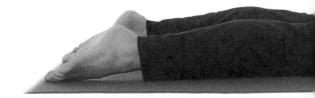

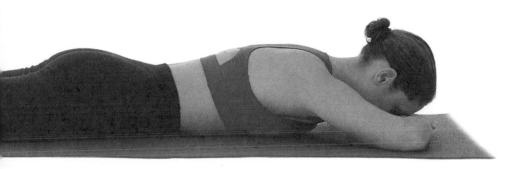

1. Lie face down, with your forehead resting on your hands and your legs extended. Relax the spine and shoulder girdle into neutral. Inhale, engaging the pelvic floor muscles and TVA.

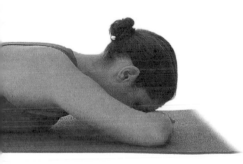

2. Exhale, and lift your left leg off the floor. Point the toes and lengthen the leg away from the body, keeping the neck long and the pelvis and ribs in alignment.

3. Inhale as you return to the start position. Repeat the movement with the right leg. Repeat the whole exercise five times, increasing to a maximum of ten.

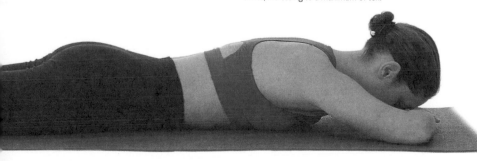

SPINE TWIST I

74

Aim: To strengthen and mobilize the spine.
Benefits: The obliques, lumbar multifidus,
transversus abdominis, and shoulder girdle.

1. Sit on the floor, with your weight evenly distributed over both
sitting bones. Extend your legs, with your inner thighs touching,
or sit in the cross-legged "tailor" position. Lengthen your spine
so that the crown of your head reaches toward the ceiling. Cross
your arms over your chest, and relax the shoulder girdle into
neutral. Inhale.

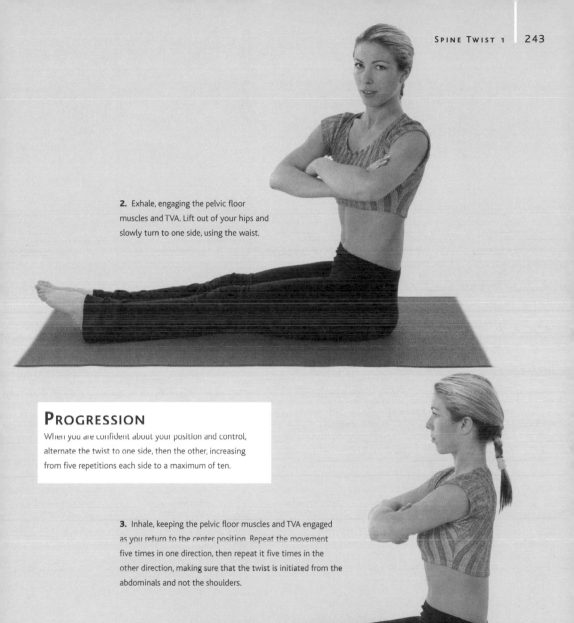

2. Exhale, engaging the pelvic floor muscles and TVA. Lift out of your hips and slowly turn to one side, using the waist.

PROGRESSION

When you are confident about your position and control, alternate the twist to one side, then the other, increasing from five repetitions each side to a maximum of ten.

3. Inhale, keeping the pelvic floor muscles and TVA engaged as you return to the center position. Repeat the movement five times in one direction, then repeat it five times in the other direction, making sure that the twist is initiated from the abdominals and not the shoulders.

75

FORWARD LEG KICK I

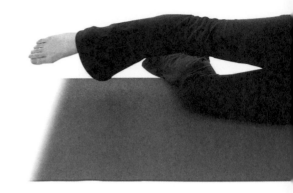

The following exercises are carried out as a series, so work through them both on one leg first, then repeat them on the other leg. Repeat each movement five times at first, gradually increasing to a maximum of ten.

Aim: To strengthen the lower back, mobilize the hips, and work the buttocks and hamstrings.

Benefits: The hip flexors, transversus abdominis, and gluteus maximus.

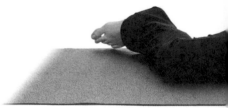

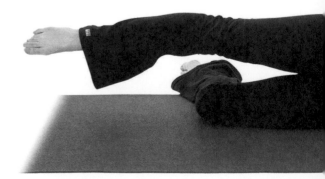

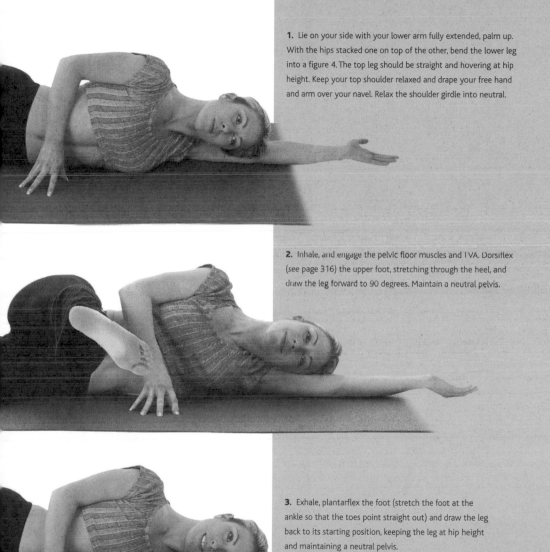

1. Lie on your side with your lower arm fully extended, palm up. With the hips stacked one on top of the other, bend the lower leg into a figure 4. The top leg should be straight and hovering at hip height. Keep your top shoulder relaxed and drape your free hand and arm over your navel. Relax the shoulder girdle into neutral.

2. Inhale, and engage the pelvic floor muscles and TVA. Dorsiflex (see page 316) the upper foot, stretching through the heel, and draw the leg forward to 90 degrees. Maintain a neutral pelvis.

3. Exhale, plantarflex the foot (stretch the foot at the ankle so that the toes point straight out) and draw the leg back to its starting position, keeping the leg at hip height and maintaining a neutral pelvis.

TOP LEG LIFT I

76

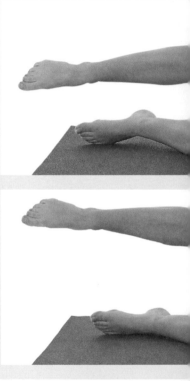

1. Lie on your side with your lower arm fully extended, palm up. With the hips stacked one on top of the other, bend the lower leg into a figure 4. The top leg should be straight and hovering at hip height. Keep your top shoulder relaxed and drape your free hand and arm over your navel. Relax the shoulder girdle into neutral.

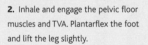

2. Inhale and engage the pelvic floor muscles and TVA. Plantarflex the foot and lift the leg slightly.

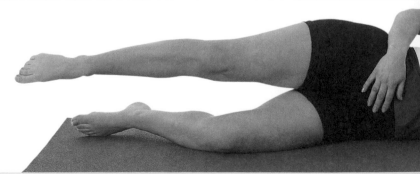

Aim: To mobilize the hips and work the buttocks and hamstrings.

Benefits: The hip flexors, transversus abdominis, gluteus maximus, and hamstrings.

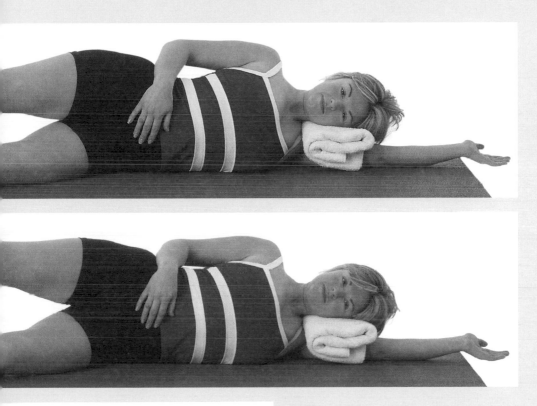

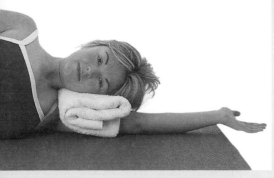

3. Exhale, and lower the leg to its starting position.

4. Repeat on the other side.

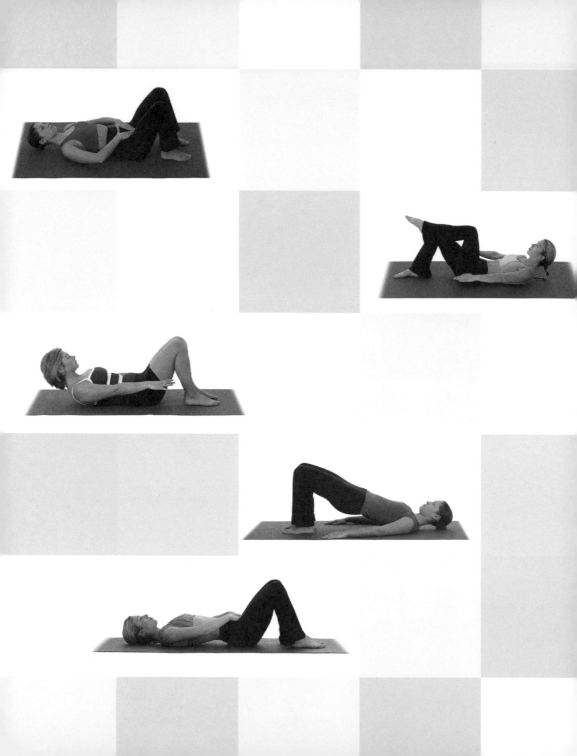

Beginner Level Exercises

INTRODUCTION

By now, you will be very familiar with the unique language of Pilates—core stability, neutral position, lateral breathing, and so on—so you are ready to move a step farther. This section contains a large number of movements from the earlier Introductory Level Exercises, but you will find that there are now subtle changes that make them a little more challenging.

Each exercise has a panel explaining the purpose of the exercise, and of the progression where relevant. For some of the exercises, you will also find tips to help you support the movement until you are ready to carry it out unaided—for example, the Abdominals 2 exercise on pages 258–259 suggests a way of lightly supporting your head until your abdominals are strong enough to take over all

the work. As always, you are not looking for instant results, so do not feel you are failing if you have to call on this extra support at first—just keep making slow and steady progress, and eventually you will find that you no longer need it.

Several of the exercises in this section also have suggestions for progressions and modifications to the basic movement. Move on to the progressions when you feel confident that you can carry out the basic move easily, or try keeping to a modification for a short while if the basic move is a little too challenging at first. Again, you are not failing if you do this—you are simply approaching the technique in the way Pilates intended and achieving quality, not quantity.

This section contains the original and best-known Pilates exercise—the One Hundred, so-called because you aim to inhale to the count of five and exhale to the count of five (making ten), then repeat the movement ten times (making the hundred). This exercise requires a very strong, stable center, along with controlled but rhythmic breathing, but the abdominal exercises will have prepared you for it.

The section ends with leg circles, a fantastic movement to finish off the leg exercises, working the hips, buttocks, and thighs and promoting mobility at the hip. To do these, the body must be very stable, and you must remember that the movement comes from the hip—do not be tempted just to wiggle your foot or toes from the ankle. What you are after is a small, very controlled movement, not huge circles—imagine your leg is inside a small pot, and you are working around the circumference. When you can perform this movement smoothly, keeping the shoulders in neutral and not allowing the body to tip either forward or back, you will know that you are well on the way to core stability.

As before, the goal of all the exercises is to start with five repetitions and build up slowly, adding one repetition at a time, until you can achieve ten repetitions in good form—that is, in a slow, controlled, flowing movement. Relax, find your rhythm, take your time and remember that focus, precision, and breathing are still all-important.

Below and opposite: This section contains movements that are a little more challenging.

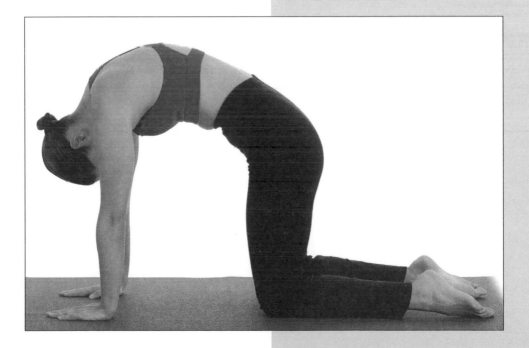

BREATHING

Aim: To strengthen the central core by activating the transversus abdominis through breathing.

Benefits: The transversus abdominis, lumbar multifidus, and pelvic floor muscles.

As with the introductory level, start with this exercise to focus your attention on your breathing.

1. Lie on your back, with your knees at 45 degrees, your feet flat on the floor, hip-width apart, and your shoulder girdle in neutral. Rest your hands across your ribcage.

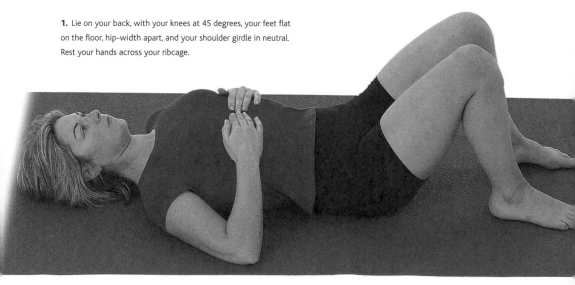

NOTE

In this exercise, it is important that you relax and observe the flow of the breath as it moves in and out of the body. To help you focus, inhale to a count of four, then exhale to a count of four.

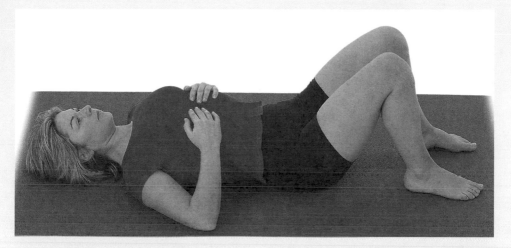

2. Inhale wide and full, feeling your ribcage expand and the
breath going into your back and sides.

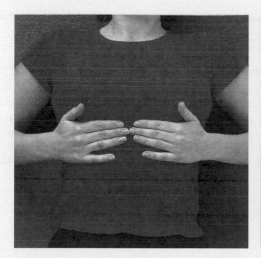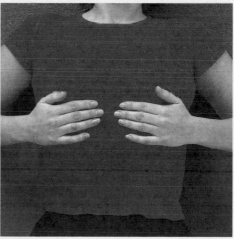

3. Exhale, gently drawing up the pelvic floor and activating the
TVA in and up (MVC 30 percent). Feel your ribcage close in and
soften, as if funneling down to the hips.

4. Continue to inhale and exhale as above, focusing your
attention on your breathing. At first, inhale and exhale five
times, increasing to a maximum of ten. Remember, your breath
is gentle, not forced. Exhale through the mouth, keeping the jaw
relaxed, and do not be tempted to blow through pursed lips.

LUMBAR ROLLS

Aim: To strengthen the central core.
Benefits: The abdominal muscles.

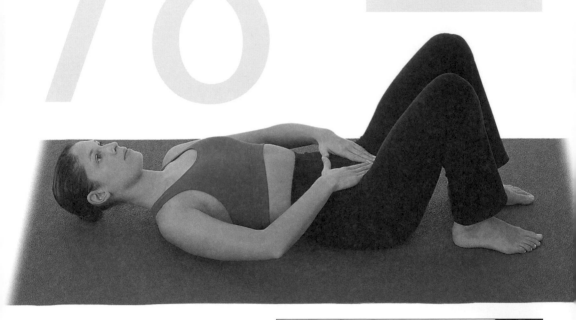

1. Lie on your back, with your knees at 45 degrees and your feet flat on the floor, hip-width apart. Place your hands on your stomach, making a triangle with your thumbs in a line at the base of your navel and your fingers splayed downward, coming together to make a point at the pubic bone (this will provide feedback as you carry out the movement). Relax your shoulder girdle and spine into neutral.

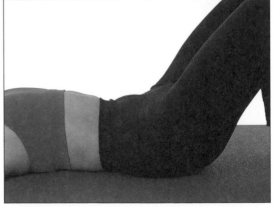

2. Inhale wide and full, feeling your ribcage expand and the breath going into your back and sides.

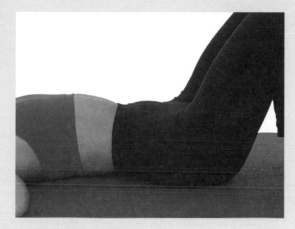

3. Exhale, engaging your pelvic floor muscles and TVA. Simultaneously, draw the pubic bone toward the navel and gently tilt the pelvis toward you, rolling your tailbone off the floor.

4. Inhale, and release the pelvis to neutral. Exhale, and arch the back gently.

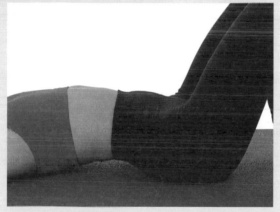

5. Inhale, and release the pelvis to neutral. Repeat the movement five times, increasing gradually to a maximum of ten.

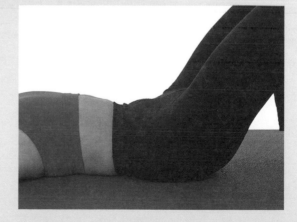

LOWER ABDOMINALS II

In the introductory level exercise for lower abdominals on pages 222–223, you held the tilt as you inhaled. Now that you are familiar with the technique, hold the contraction—NOT YOUR BREATH—for ten to 20 seconds as you inhale and exhale rhythmically.

Aim: To strengthen the central core.
Benefits: The lower abdominal muscles.

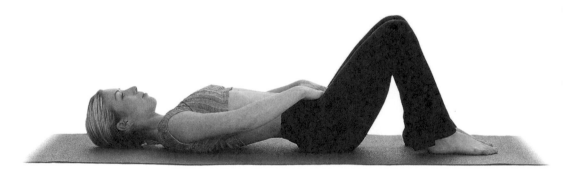

1. Lie on your back, with your knees at 45 degrees and your feet flat on the floor, hip-width apart. Either rest your arms at your sides, palms down, or lay your hands in a triangle on your stomach as in the previous exercise. Relax your shoulder girdle and spine into neutral.

2. Inhale, wide and full.

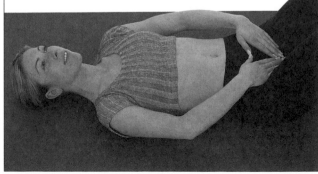

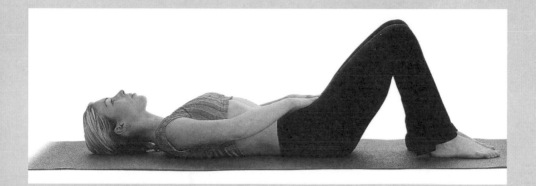

3. Exhale. Simultaneously, draw the pubic bone toward the navel and, using your abdominals to initiate the movement, gently tilt the pelvis toward you.

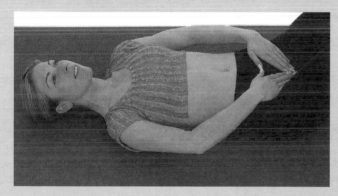

4. Inhale, and hold the tilt, keeping the TVA contraction activated at 30 percent as you breathe rhythmically for ten to 20 seconds.

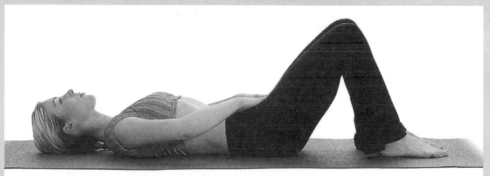

5. Exhale as you roll back to neutral. Repeat the movement five times, gradually increasing to a maximum of ten.

ABDOMINALS II

80

In the introductory level exercise for the abdominals on pages 224–225, you held the flexion as you inhaled. In this exercise, you release the flexion by five percent as you inhale, and come back to it as you exhale, without touching the floor. Keep your gaze on your knees as you carry out the movement to ensure good head and neck placement. If you feel your head getting heavy, support it lightly with one hand, your elbow open wide like a wing—but do not clamp your head too hard or draw it forward.

Aim: To flex the spine while strengthening and stabilizing the central core.
Benefits: The neck, shoulders, spine, and abdominals.

1. Lie on your back, with your knees at 45 degrees and your feet in line with your knees, hip-width apart. Rest your arms by your sides, palms down. Lengthen your neck, and relax your upper body, keeping your shoulder girdle neutral.

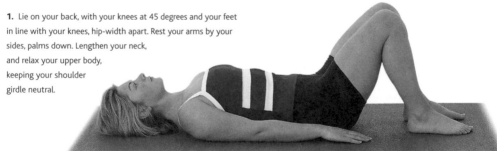

2. Inhale, and lengthen through the back of your neck by slightly nodding your chin to your chest, without raising your head.

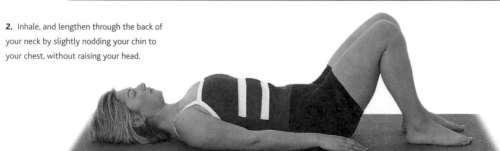

3. Exhale, and flex forward, allowing your head and shoulders to curl off the floor and bringing the ribcage toward the pelvis. Raise your arms off the floor, level with your shoulders. Make sure your pelvic floor muscles and TVA are engaged, navel to spine, and that your spine remains neutral.

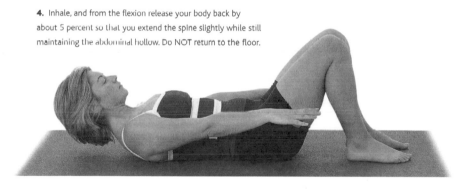

4. Inhale, and from the flexion release your body back by about 5 percent so that you extend the spine slightly while still maintaining the abdominal hollow. Do NOT return to the floor.

5. Exhale, drawing up the pelvic floor and contracting the navel to spine by five percent so that you are scooped as in Step 3. Repeat the movement five times, gradually increasing to a maximum of ten.

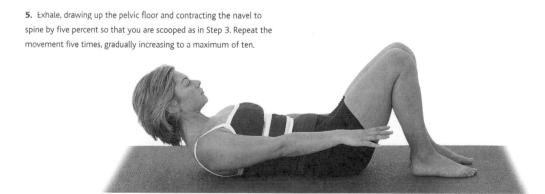

ONE HUNDRED

This is perhaps the best known of the Pilates movements, combining the main aims of Pilates—to strengthen and stabilize the central core while promoting controlled and rhythmic breathing. Mastering the Abdominals 1 and 2 movements will prepare you well for this exercise. In its most advanced form, the One Hundred includes gentle beats with the arms, but for stability the arms are kept strong but static here.

Aim: To flex the spine, stabilize the shoulder girdle and pelvis, strengthen the central core, and promote breath control.
Benefits: The neck, shoulders, spine, abdominals, and breathing.

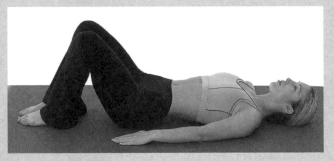

1. Lie on your back, with your knees at 45 degrees, your feet flat on the floor, and your inner thighs connected. Rest your arms by your sides, palms down, but keep them strong, with a slight bend in the elbows. Relax the shoulder girdle into neutral. Inhale, and lengthen through the back of the neck.

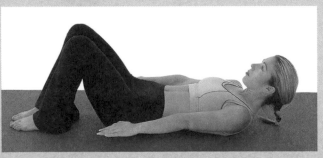

2. Exhale, and flex forward, allowing your head and shoulders to curl off the floor and bringing the ribcage toward the pelvis. Raise your arms off the floor and keep them strong, level with your shoulders. Make sure your pelvic floor muscles and TVA are engaged, navel to spine, and that your spine remains neutral.

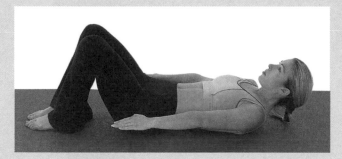

3. Inhale, and count to five, maintaining the TVA contraction at 20–30 percent.

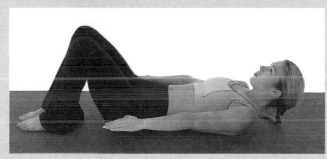

4. Exhale, and count to five, holding the flexion and pulling the contraction to 30 percent. Repeat the movement five times, gradually increasing to a maximum of ten. With each repetition, try to maintain the center connection and not allow the major abdominal muscle to dome.

PROGRESSION

Only try these variations once you are confident of your stability, as you MUST be able to keep your pelvis and spine in neutral, without arching or straining the lower back or lifting the hips.

1. Raise one foot so that the knee is at 90 degrees, directly over the hip. To do this, inhale and roll your pelvis as in Lower Abdominals 2 (page 256), then exhale and raise one leg as in Knee Folds (page 228).

2. Raise both feet so that both knees are at 90 degrees, directly over the hip. To do this, first raise one leg as above, then inhale, maintaining the position, and exhale as you raise the other leg.

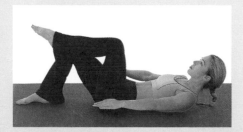

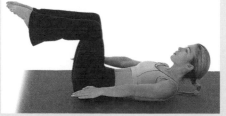

BENT KNEE CIRCLE

82

This is a fantastic exercise for mobilizing the hip joints, and is particularly useful if you spend a lot of time sitting down or driving, when the muscles of the hip and inner thighs get very little stretch. When circling the knees, make sure you exhale when the leg is moving away from you, because this is when you most need stability and a good connection with the center. In its most advanced form, this movement is carried out with the leg fully extended.

Aim: To mobilize the hip joint and stretch the muscles of the hip and inner thigh.
Benefits: The abdomen, hips, and inner thighs.

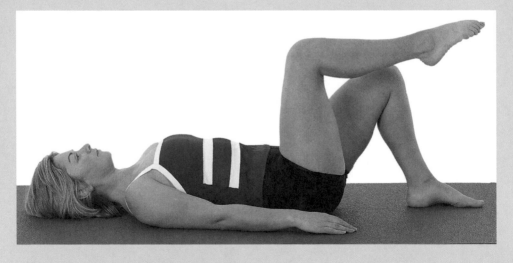

1. Lie on your back, with your knees bent at 45 degrees and your feet flat on the floor, hip-width apart. Rest your arms by your sides, palms down, or place them on your stomach in a triangle for feedback—the sides of the triangle should remain even as you carry out the movement. Relax your shoulder girdle and spine into neutral. Inhale. Exhale, engaging the pelvic floor muscles and TVA, and take one knee up to 90 degrees, in line with the hip. Hold the position.

2. Inhale, keeping the pelvic floor muscles and TVA engaged. Circle the knee clockwise toward you to the midline, keeping the leg stationary—imagine you are stirring the leg in the hip socket.

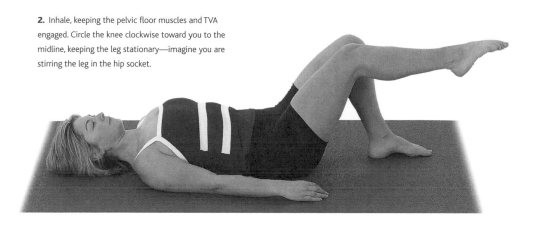

3. Exhale, completing the circle by taking the knee away from you. Continue, circling the knee five times clockwise and five times anticlockwise. Repeat the movement with the other leg.

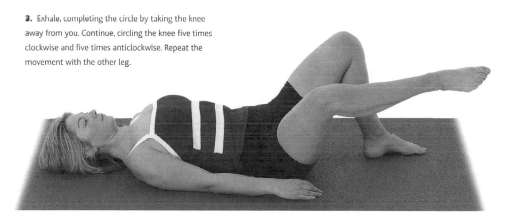

PROGRESSION

Take both knees to 90 degrees, and place your fingers on your kneecaps. This time, create only small circles, using your fingers to give you feedback that your legs are moving evenly. When circling both legs like this, it is essential to keep the pelvis stable so that the back does not arch off the floor.

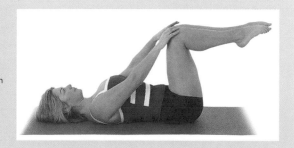

ROLLING

83

Aim: Abdominal connection and spinal articulation, stretch of the erector spine muscles.
Benefits: The spine, neck, shoulders, and abdominals.

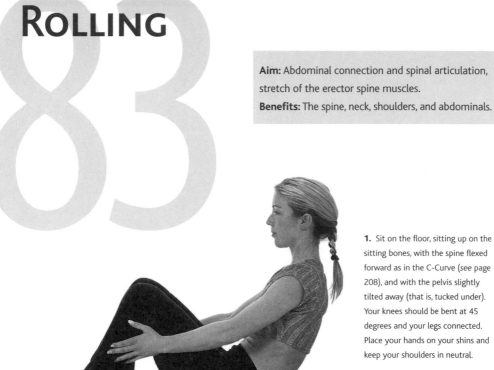

1. Sit on the floor, sitting up on the sitting bones, with the spine flexed forward as in the C-Curve (*see* page 208), and with the pelvis slightly tilted away (that is, tucked under). Your knees should be bent at 45 degrees and your legs connected. Place your hands on your shins and keep your shoulders in neutral.

2. Inhale. Follow your pelvic tilt and C-Curve by rolling back to the floor behind you.

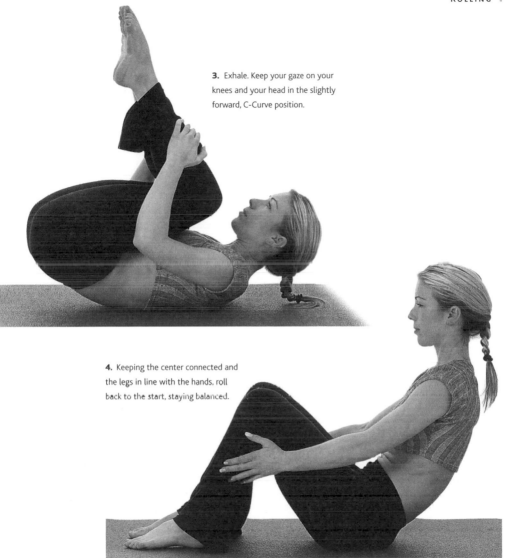

3. Exhale. Keep your gaze on your knees and your head in the slightly forward, C-Curve position.

4. Keeping the center connected and the legs in line with the hands, roll back to the start, staying balanced.

VARIATION

As a variation, try placing your palms on your calves instead of your shins. You may find that this releases the tension on your shoulder muscles, enabling you to relax them and to avoid shrugging up. While learning this exercise, you can also place your feet down between each roll.

SINGLE LEG STRETCH

84

This exercise is a more challenging progression of the sliding leg movement on pages 226–227. Start slowly, keeping the body flat and the legs at 90 degrees. Stretch your legs out at a pace that allows you to keep your body in neutral. As you gain strength and control over the central core, flex the body before stretching out the legs.

Aim: To promote coordination, to strengthen and stabilize the abdominals, and to stretch the leg muscles.
Benefits: The neck, shoulders, transversus abdominis, hip flexors (eccentrically), and hip extensors and quadriceps (concentrically).

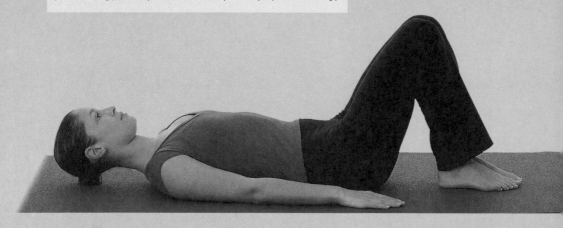

1. Lie on your back, with your inner thighs connected, your knees bent at 45 degrees and your feet flat on the floor. Rest your arms by your sides with your palms down and a slight bend in your elbows. Inhale, lengthening through the back of the neck.

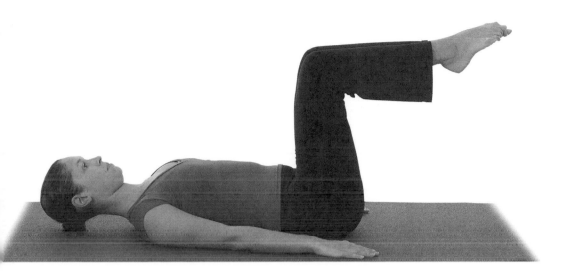

2. Exhale, and initiate the pelvic tilt, engaging the pelvic floor muscles and the TVA, navel to spine, and keeping the spine neutral. Keeping the inner thighs connected, raise both knees to 90 degrees. Inhale, maintaining the position.

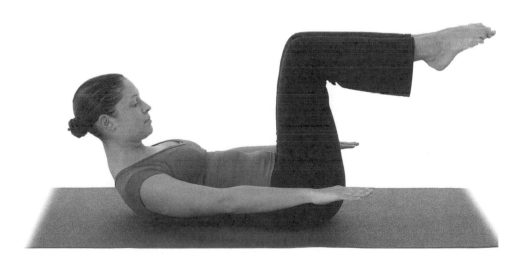

3. Exhale and flex forward, allowing the head and shoulders to curl off the floor and bringing the ribcage toward the pelvis. Raise your arms to shoulder level. Keep the pelvic floor muscles and TVA engaged, navel to spine, and neutral spine. Inhale, to prepare.

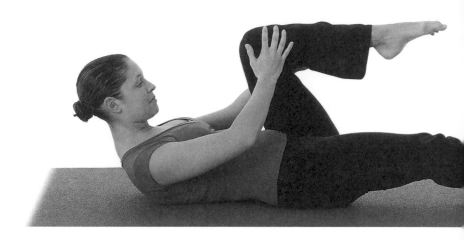

4. Exhale, stretching one leg away from the body but maintaining the TVA contraction.

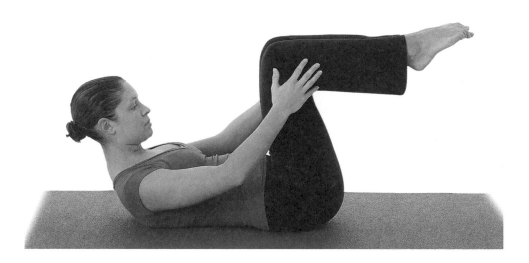

5. Inhale, returning the leg to center.

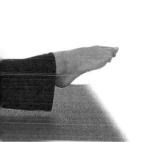

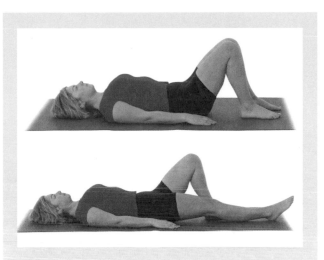

MODIFICATIONS

If you are unable to perform this exercise, substitute the leg slides from the Introductory level on pages 226–227, then carry on with the remainder of the exercises from this level.

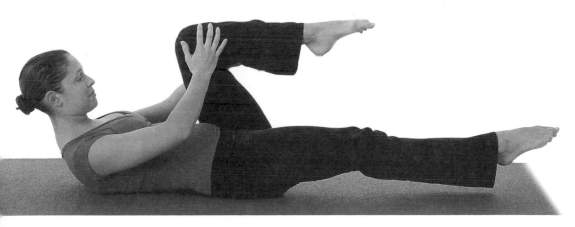

6. Exhale, stretching the other leg away from the body. Repeat the exercise five times in a cycling movement, gradually increasing to a maximum of ten.

DOUBLE LEG STRETCH

85

This movement requires a very strong and stable central core, especially as you progress. You can raise one leg at a time or both together, depending on your level of stability.

Aim: To promote coordination, to strengthen and stabilize the abdominals, and to stretch the leg muscles.
Benefits: The transversus abdominis, pectorals, and hip flexors (eccentrically and concentrically).

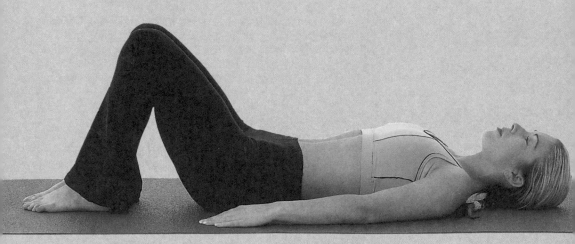

1. Lie on your back, with your inner thighs connected, your knees bent at 45 degrees and your feet flat on the floor, hip-width apart. Rest your arms by your sides with your palms down and a slight bend in your elbows. Inhale, and lengthen through the cervical spine.

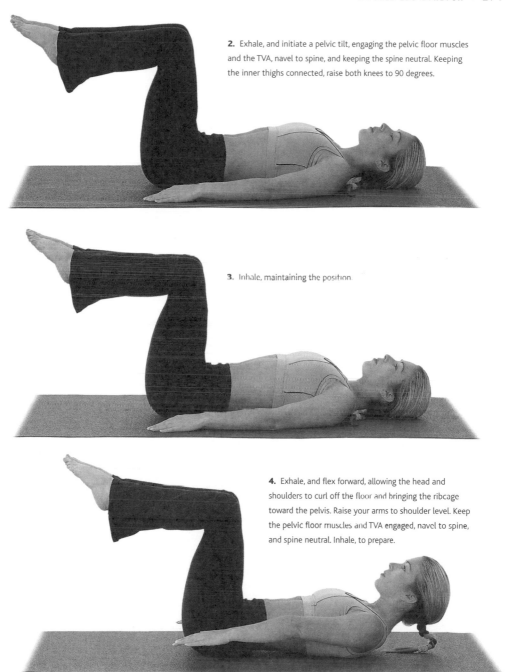

2. Exhale, and initiate a pelvic tilt, engaging the pelvic floor muscles and the TVA, navel to spine, and keeping the spine neutral. Keeping the inner thighs connected, raise both knees to 90 degrees.

3. Inhale, maintaining the position.

4. Exhale, and flex forward, allowing the head and shoulders to curl off the floor and bringing the ribcage toward the pelvis. Raise your arms to shoulder level. Keep the pelvic floor muscles and TVA engaged, navel to spine, and spine neutral. Inhale, to prepare.

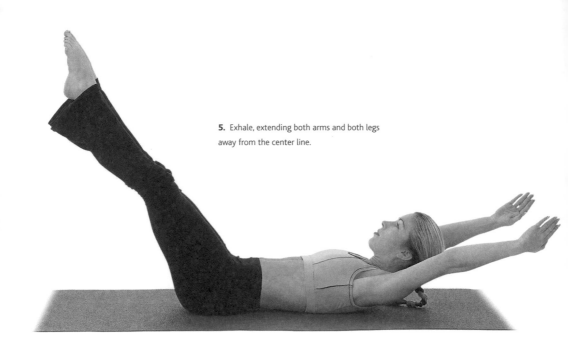

5. Exhale, extending both arms and both legs away from the center line.

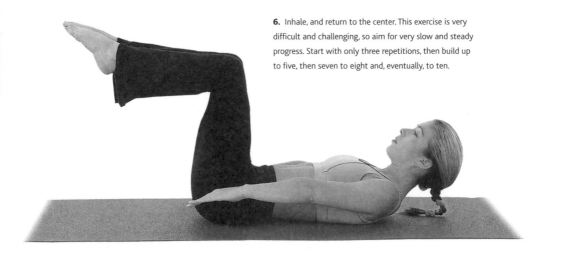

6. Inhale, and return to the center. This exercise is very difficult and challenging, so aim for very slow and steady progress. Start with only three repetitions, then build up to five, then seven to eight and, eventually, to ten.

MODIFICATIONS

When carrying out the modifications, flex the upper body off the floor and make sure you have a very strong, connected center. Inhale and circle your arms to the ceiling, then exhale as you draw the shoulder blades down your back, completing the circle. The arms must be strong like beating wings, but not tense. Your shoulders and the shoulder girdle must be stable, with the blades being drawn down as you lower the arms. This will enable you to circle (circumduct) your arms in the optimum position, without causing tension in the neck or shoulder area.

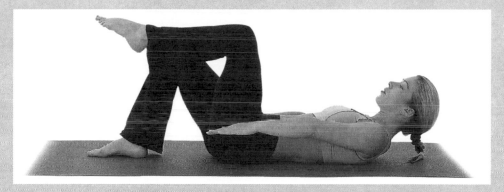

1. Flex the upper body and circle the arms from the shoulders. Keep the arms firm from shoulder to finger. Keep the knees bent at 90 degrees, or leave one at 45 degrees and bend the other to 90 degrees.

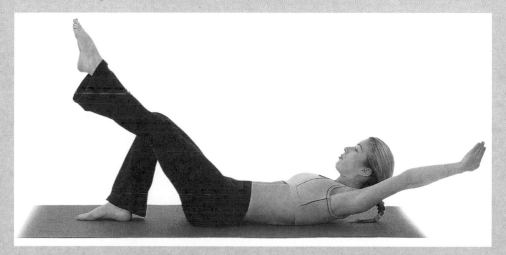

2. Continue as steps 2 to 4 (*see* page 271). However, in Step 5, only extend the arm and leg on one side at a time.

SHOULDER BRIDGE

86

This is an ideal exercise for rolling away the stresses of the day. It is not a pelvic thrust—the aim is to roll through the spine, segment by segment. Roll only as far as you are comfortable each time, starting with the lower abdomen, then progressing to the navel, the ribcage, and, eventually, to the base of the shoulder blades. At the top of the position the shoulder blades must be relaxed.

Aim: To lengthen the body and articulate through the spine.
Benefits: The transversus abdominis, the gluteus maximus, and the hamstrings.

1. Lie on your back, with your knees at 45 degrees and your feet hip-width apart. Rest your arms by your sides, palms down. Lengthen your neck, and relax your upper body, keeping your shoulder girdle neutral. Inhale.

2. Exhale, and initiate the pelvic tilt toward the ribcage, engaging the pelvic floor muscles, TVA, and navel to spine and keeping the spine in neutral. Articulate through the spine from the tailbone, one vertebra at a time, as far as the base of the shoulder blades, so that your body forms a bridge shape. Do not roll as far as the neck (cervical spine). Inhale, maintaining the TVA contraction.

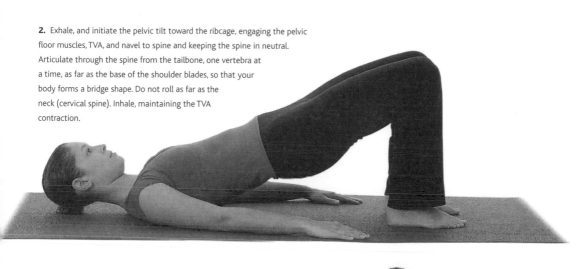

3. Exhale and articulate, one vertebra at a time, back to the start position, dropping the heart first, rolling into the navel and lastly dropping the tailbone.

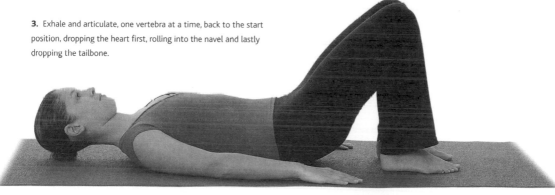

4. Repeat the movement five times, gradually increasing to a maximum of ten.

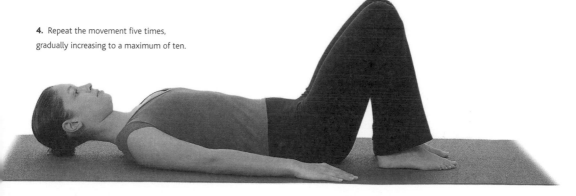

SPINE STRETCH II

This movement is the same as in the Introductory Level (*see* pages 238–239). However, it is essential to do this exercise at this stage, as the body needs to flex forward to balance the muscle work.

Aim: To strengthen the abdominals and lengthen the muscles of the spine.
Benefits: The abdominals, spine, and hips.

1. Sit on the floor, with your weight evenly distributed over both sitting bones and your spine in neutral. Lengthen your spine so that the top of your head reaches toward the ceiling. Extend your legs, hip-width apart (if your hamstrings feel too tight in this position, bend your knees slightly or sit on a rolled towel or mat). Extend your arms in front of you, slightly below shoulder level, with the palms facing up to help the shoulders stay relaxed and stable. Relax the shoulder girdle into neutral.

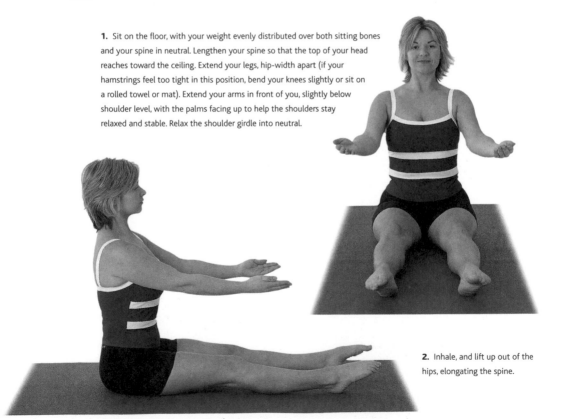

2. Inhale, and lift up out of the hips, elongating the spine.

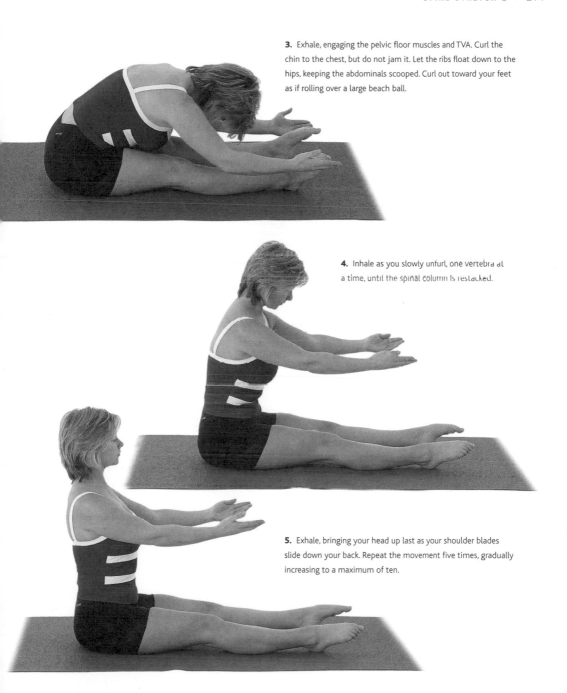

3. Exhale, engaging the pelvic floor muscles and TVA. Curl the chin to the chest, but do not jam it. Let the ribs float down to the hips, keeping the abdominals scooped. Curl out toward your feet as if rolling over a large beach ball.

4. Inhale as you slowly unfurl, one vertebra at a time, until the spinal column is restacked.

5. Exhale, bringing your head up last as your shoulder blades slide down your back. Repeat the movement five times, gradually increasing to a maximum of ten.

SPINE TWIST II

88

This is another lovely, relaxing exercise. Imagine yourself as a corkscrew, exhaling as you draw up and twist, and inhaling as you unwind back to the center, maintaining the connection.

At first, work one side at a time, keeping the pace even and making sure the seat bones are even and remain on the floor. As you progress, you can work from one side to the other in a flowing movement. A further progression is to hold the twist on the exhale, then push round a little farther before inhaling and returning to the center in one movement.

1. Sit on the floor, with your weight evenly distributed over both sitting bones and your spine in neutral. Lengthen your spine so that the top of your head reaches toward the ceiling. Extend your legs, keeping the inner thighs connected (if your hamstrings feel too tight in this position, bend your knees slightly or sit on a rolled towel or mat). Extend the arms laterally, palms up. Relax the shoulder girdle into neutral. Inhale.

Aim: To work the muscles at the waistline (obliques) and the spine rotators.
Benefits: The obliques, lumbar multifidus, transversus abdominis, and shoulder girdle.

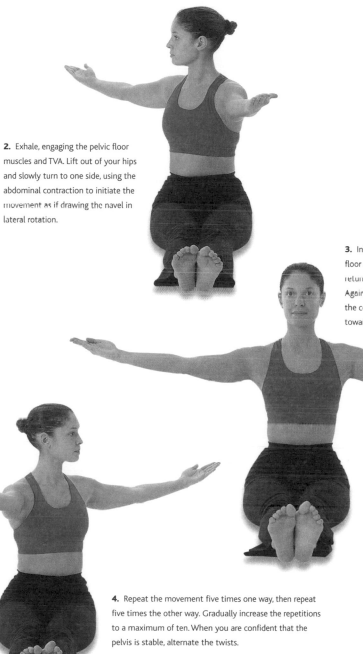

2. Exhale, engaging the pelvic floor muscles and TVA. Lift out of your hips and slowly turn to one side, using the abdominal contraction to initiate the movement as if drawing the navel in lateral rotation.

3. Inhale, maintaining the pelvic floor and TVA contraction as you return to the center position. Again, initiate the movement from the center as if drawing the navel toward the midline.

4. Repeat the movement five times one way, then repeat five times the other way. Gradually increase the repetitions to a maximum of ten. When you are confident that the pelvis is stable, alternate the twists.

SWAN DIVE II

Positioning your hands at shoulder level in the progression exercise will help stabilize you and enable you to peel your upper body farther off the floor, but maintain control in the center and resist the temptation to push up on your hands. The shoulders must stay in neutral and the ribs and pelvis must remain integrated to ensure that the ribs do not move forward, taking the abdominals with them.

Aim: To strengthen and stabilize the shoulder girdle and spine.
Benefits: The shoulders, spine, transversus abdominis, hamstrings, and gluteus maximus.

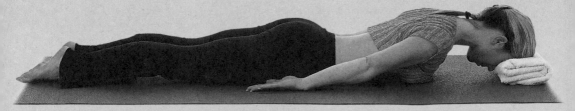

1. Lie face down, with your forehead resting on the floor on a folded towel or soft pillow. Rest your arms by your sides, palms facing out, and relax your shoulders into neutral. Keep your inner thighs connected and your toes pointed. Inhale. Exhale, engaging the pelvic floor muscles and TVA and lengthening through the spine.

2. Inhale, peeling your upper body off the floor from the hips. Lengthen through the back, pulling your shoulder blades down. Keep the abdominals engaged for support. Keep the chest wide open and the shoulders in neutral. Keep your eyes focused on the floor and do not push back the neck and head.

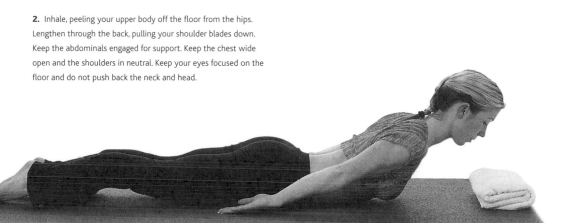

3. Exhale, maintaining the connection with the center, and lower the body to the floor. Repeat the movement five times, gradually increasing to a maximum of ten.

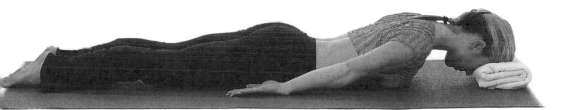

PROGRESSION

1. When you have achieved good form working the upper body, extend both arms together, with the shoulder blades relaxed and in neutral.

2. Combine the arm and leg movements, lifting and extending the right arm and leg together, followed by the left arm and leg.

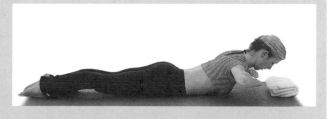

3. Combine the arm and leg movements, lifting and extending the right arm and left leg together, followed by the left arm and right leg.

SWIMMING II

If you have a back or hip problem, seek advice before attempting this exercise, as bilateral movement can exacerbate some conditions. Take the exercise slowly, as it requires good central stability while the arms and legs are pulling away from each other. The progression exercises will promote coordination and movement integration. Your eventual aim is to extend the arms and legs from the center and beat them up and down in a swimming motion, as you inhale and exhale rhythmically.

Aim: To lengthen the spine and strengthen and stabilize the center.

Benefits: The transversus abdominis, shoulder stabilizers, and spine extensors.

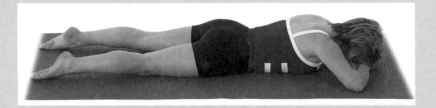

1. Lie face down, with your forehead resting on your hands and your legs relaxed, hip-width apart. Relax the spine and shoulder girdle into neutral. Inhale, engaging the pelvic floor muscles and TVA.

2. Exhale, and lift your left leg off the floor. Point the toes and lengthen the leg away from the body, keeping the neck long and the pelvis and ribs in alignment.

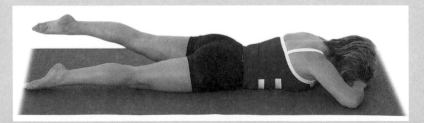

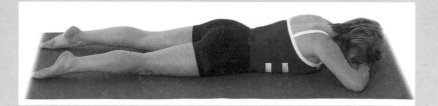

3. Inhale as you return to the start position. Repeat the movement five times with the left leg, then five times with the right leg. Gradually increase the repetitions to ten. When you feel confident that your legs and pelvis are stable, alternate the legs for a total of six to ten repetitions (that is, raising each leg three to five times). Inhale, engaging the pelvic floor muscles and TVA.

4. Exhale, and extend the right arm in front of you, off the floor. Keep your head in line with your arm, your shoulder blades melting down your back and your neck long—focus your gaze on the floor. There should be no tension in the upper body—as you extend one arm, keep the other arm folded as shown to aid stability.

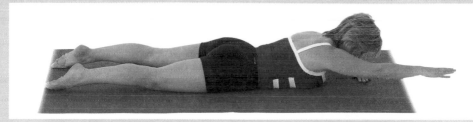

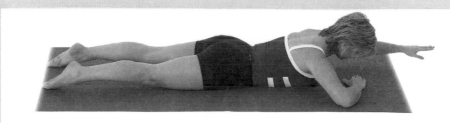

5. Inhale as you return to the start position. Repeat the movement five times with the right arm, then five times with the left arm. Gradually increase the repetitions to ten. When you feel confident that your arms and shoulders are stable, alternate the arms for a total of six to ten repetitions (that is, raising each arm three to five times).

PROGRESSION

1. When you have achieved good form with both the legs and the arms, combine the two movements, lifting the right arm and leg together, followed by the left arm and leg.

2. Combine the two movements, lifting the right arm and left leg, followed by the left arm and right leg.

CAT STRETCH II

91

Maintain the connection to the center throughout this exercise. When you return the spine to the start position, do not let it drop or sag toward the floor—imagine yourself supporting a tray on a flat back, with the shoulders set, the head and neck in line with the spine, and the pelvis in neutral.

Aim: To mobilize the spine and help with stabilization.
Benefits: The spine, shoulders, neck, and abdomen.

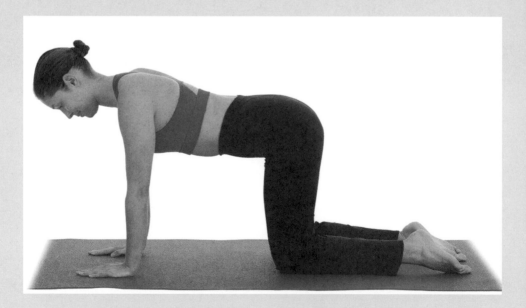

1. Kneel on all fours, with your spine and shoulder girdle in neutral, your knees under your hips, and your hands under your shoulders. Inhale and, keeping the body in neutral, engage the pelvic floor muscles and TVA.

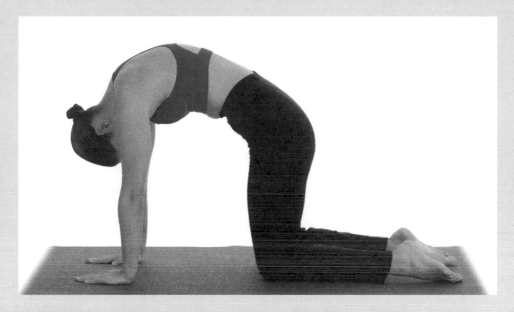

2. Exhale and, keeping the abdominals scooped to the spine for support, flex the spine, curling from the tailbone toward the head and dropping your head between your arms. Inhale at the top of the movement and extend the spine so your back is arched like a cat stretching. Maintain the TVA contraction.

3. Exhale and uncurl the spine from the tailbone, allowing the head to come back up to the start position. Repeat the movement five times, gradually increasing to a maximum of ten.

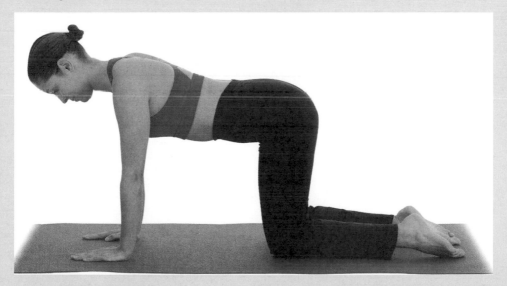

FORWARD LEG KICK II

92

For this exercise, the center needs to be really strong as the base of support is limited and the body will be inclined either to roll forward or rock back. So, although it is a leg exercise, keep thinking "center." You may find it helpful to place a small towel between your arm and your head for support—this will help to keep your neck in alignment with the spine.

Aim: To strengthen and stabilize the center and work the hips and abdomen.
Benefits: The hips, flexors, transversus abdominis, and gluteus maximus.

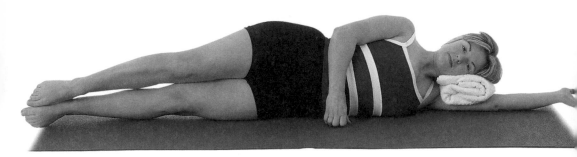

1. Lie on your side, with your hips stacked one on top of the other and your legs together with the inner thighs connected. Extend your lower arm, palm up, so that you are in a straight line from your fingertips to your toes. Now angle your legs forward slightly, without changing the position of your spine, which must still be in a straight line from your head to your tailbone.

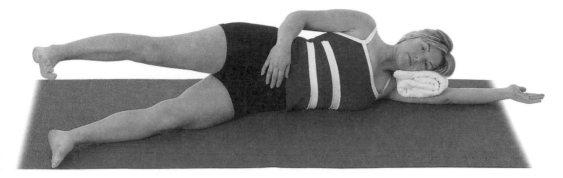

2. From this position, separate the top leg and bring it back in line with your hip joint, hovering at hip height, with the foot dorsiflexed (bent). Keep the knee facing forward in the same direction as the hip—do not let it rotate toward the floor. Bend the upper arm at the elbow with the palm over your stomach, for feedback. Keep the top shoulder relaxed and in alignment, and the shoulder girdle in neutral. Rest your head on your arm to keep in line with the spine.

3. Inhale, engaging the pelvic floor muscles and TVA. With the foot dorsiflexed, stretch through the heel. Draw the leg forward to 90 degrees, maintaining a neutral pelvis—you may not be able to achieve the 90 degrees at first, so go as far as you can without losing form and progress gradually.

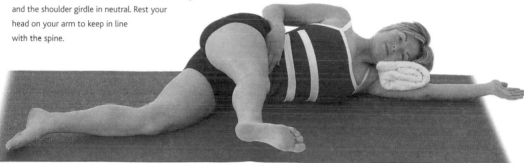

4. Exhale, plantarflex (stretch) the foot and draw the leg back to the start position, maintaining a neutral pelvis and keeping the leg at hip height. Repeat the movement five times with one leg, then turn over and work the other leg. Gradually increase the repetitions to a maximum of ten.

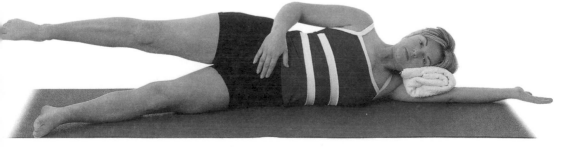

93

TOP LEG LIFT II

As with the previous exercise, the center needs to be really strong as the base of support is limited and the body will be inclined either to roll forward or rock back. So, although it is a leg exercise, keep thinking "center."

Aim: To strengthen and stabilize the center, and work the hips, abdomen, hamstrings, and calves.
Benefits: Abductors of the buttocks and top leg, and transversus abdominis.

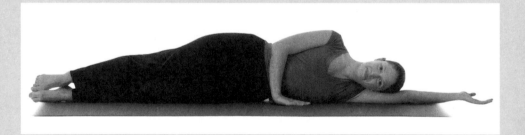

1. Lie on your side, with your hips stacked one on top of the other and your legs together with the inner thigh connected. Extend your lower arm, palm up, so that you are in a straight line from your fingertips to your toes. Now angle your legs forward slightly, without changing the position of your spine, which must still be in a straight line from your head to your tailbone.

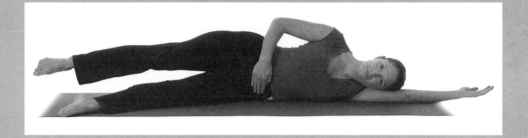

2. From this position, separate the top leg and bring it back in line with your hip joint, hovering at hip height. Point your toes. Keep the knee facing forward in the same direction as the hip—do not let it rotate toward the floor. Bend the upper arm at the elbow with the palm over your stomach, for feedback. Keep the top shoulder relaxed and in alignment, and the shoulder girdle in neutral (not rounded either forward or back). Rest your head on your arm to keep in line with the spine.

3. Inhale, engaging the pelvic floor muscles and TVA. Keeping the toes pointed, slowly lift the leg up from the hip to a maximum of 25 degrees. Lengthen through the toes, as if reaching for a light switch.

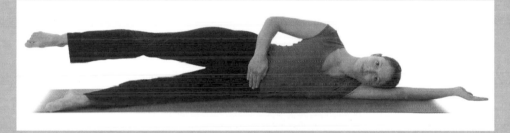

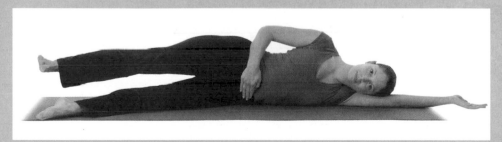

4. Exhale, and at the top of the movement draw the toes toward you as you lower the leg back to the start position, lengthening through the heel as if pressing the foot into a stirrup. Repeat the movement five times, keeping the leg and foot movement flowing—do not pause at the top or bottom of the movement—then turn over and work the other leg. Gradually increase the repetitions to a maximum of ten.

CIRCLES

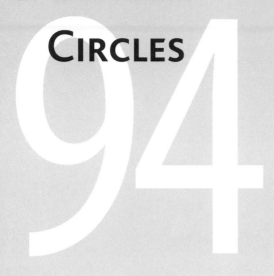

This movement is an excellent way to finish the leg series exercises. As with the previous exercises, the center needs to be really strong as the base of support is limited and the body will be inclined either to roll forward or rock back. Make sure you are drawing the circles from your hip, not simply wiggling your foot or toes.

Aim: To work the hips, buttocks, and thighs and promote hip mobility.
Benefits: Transversus abdominis and hip mobility.

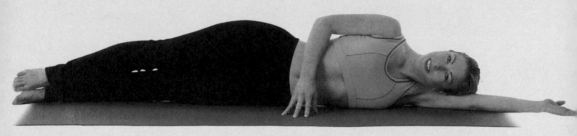

1. Lie on your side, with your hips stacked one on top of the other and your legs together, with the inner thighs connected. Extend your lower arm, palm up, so that you are in a straight line from your fingertips to your toes. Now angle your legs forward slightly, without changing the position of your spine, which must still be in a straight line from your head to your tail.

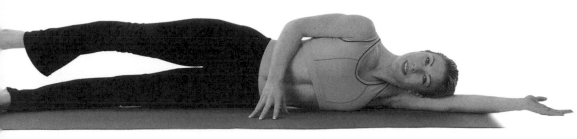

2. From this position, separate the top leg and bring it back in line with your hip joint, hovering at hip height. Point your toes. Keep the knee facing forward in the same direction as the hip—do not let it rotate toward the floor. Bend the upper arm at the elbow with the palm over your stomach, for feedback. Keep the top shoulder relaxed and in alignment, and the shoulder girdle in neutral (not rounded either forward or back). Rest your head on your arm to keep in line with the spine. Inhale, wide and full, engaging the pelvic floor muscles and TVA.

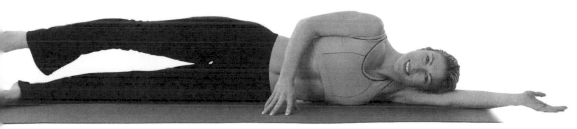

3. Exhale, and draw circles with your leg—five to the front and five back. Keep the circles small—imagine that your leg is inside a small pot, and that you are working around the circumference of the pot. Repeat the movement five times, then turn over and work the other leg. Gradually increase the repetitions to a maximum of ten.

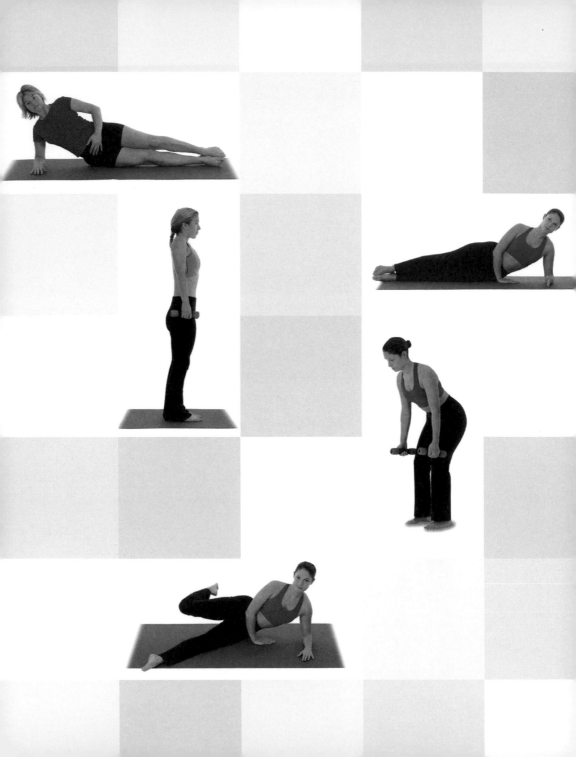

ADVANCED PILATES

INTRODUCTION

This small batch of advanced-level exercises really is quite challenging, but you have been very well prepared for them in the earlier levels, so think positively—you can do it! Do not move on to these until you feel really confident that you are ready, however, and when you do, approach them in exactly the same way as before. Make slow but steady progress and focus all your attention on each movement. There is a lot going on here, so you will need all your concentration, as well as controlled, rhythmic breathing.

For the leg exercises, your base of support is now very limited—whereas in earlier levels you have had the lower leg bent to help hold you in place, here the leg is only slightly angled. This means that if your shoulders and pelvis are not maintained in the neutral position, and your central core is not strong and stable, you are very likely to tip backward or forward. You are also incorporating a side bend into the movement, so you need to be careful not to allow the ribs to sink or collapse toward the floor. Resting your fingertips very lightly on the floor will give you excellent feedback—as soon as you feel any pressure on them, it is an indication that you are not holding the essential strong line through the body from pelvis to shoulder.

There are two advanced arm exercises in this section for working the biceps and triceps—great for toning up flab. As with the leg exercises, it is important that you really control the movement of the arms—do not swing them up and down wildly, but imagine instead that you are working against

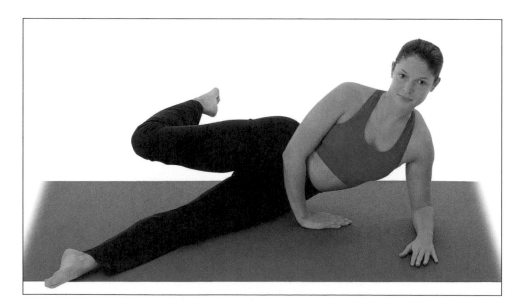

flowing water, offering that gentle resistance. The movements are more effective if you add weight, either by wearing a pair of professional hand weights on your wrists, or by holding a can of soup or beans in each hand—just make sure the contents are the same weight.

This section includes the ultimate Pilates move—the Advanced One Hundred (*see* pages 310–311), which pulls together the abdominal exercises, the lumbar roll, and the knee folds, along with superb breath control. You will have a great sense of achievement when you can do this exercise, because it is very demanding of every part of the body but most particularly of the central core, which must be 100 percent stable to support you to a count of ten as you flex the upper body and extend both legs toward the ceiling without any shuddering or loss of form or breath control.

Sounds out of your reach? Of course not! You will get there, although it may take some time unless you were already very fit to start with, and even then you may have to rationalize some of your earlier training. But just imagine—when you can do this exercise, you really will be ready to take on the world! Just keep those Pilates principles in mind—breathing, control, and concentration; precision, relaxation, and alignment; motivation and visualization—and do the best that you can.

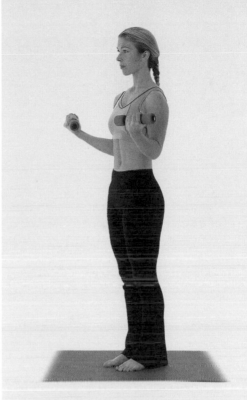

Above, below, and opposite: Make slow but steady progress and focus all your attention on each movement.

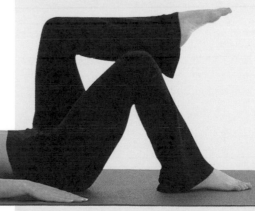

SIDE BICYCLE

95

The leg exercises in the earlier sections can be made more advanced by adopting this side-bend position of the body. It is very important that when you are in the side-bend position you do not let the ribs sink or collapse to the floor. Keep the ribs connected to a strong center, so that your body is strong from the pelvis to the shoulder.

Aim: To strengthen and mobilize the hips and work the buttocks and hamstrings.
Benefits: The hips, gluteus maximus, and hamstrings.

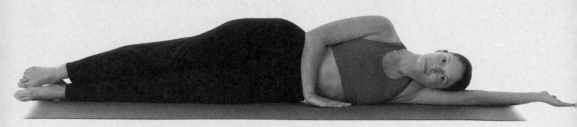

1. Lie on your side, with your hips stacked one on top of the other and your legs together with the inner thighs connected. Extend your lower arm, palm up, so that you are in a straight line from your fingertips to your toes. Keep your head in line with your spine, with your chin forward. Inhale, and as you do so place the palm of your upper hand on the floor to aid in pressing you up.

2. Exhale, and draw your lower arm in toward your body, placing the elbow directly under your shoulder and the forearm on its side, with the fingers pointed away from the body. Keep the top shoulder in neutral, and rest the arm across the navel with the hand (or fingertips as you become more proficient) on the floor for balance.

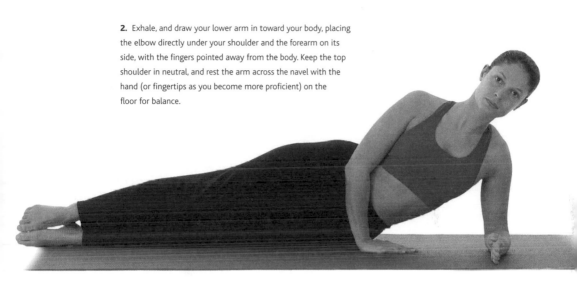

3. Now angle your legs forward slightly, without changing the position of your spine, which must still be in a straight line from your head to your tail. From this position, separate the top leg and bring it back in line with your hip joint, hovering at hip height. Point your toes. Keep the knee facing forward in the same direction as the hip—do not let it rotate toward the floor.

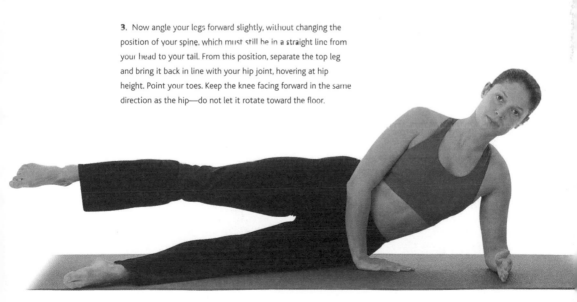

4. With the top leg hovering at hip height, inhale as you bend the working leg back with the heel toward your buttocks.

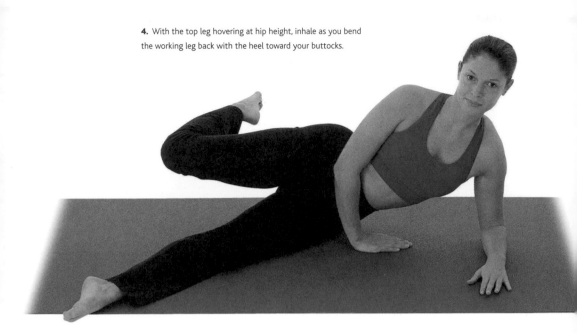

5. Extend the leg forward with the knee at 90 degrees.

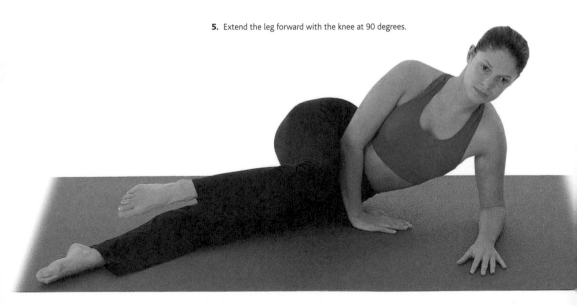

6. Repeat the movement five times, keeping the leg and foot movement flowing—do not pause. Keep the center connected, as the body will tend to rock forward with the weight of the extended leg. Turn over and work the other leg, repeating the movement five times. Gradually increase the repetitions to a maximum of ten on each leg.

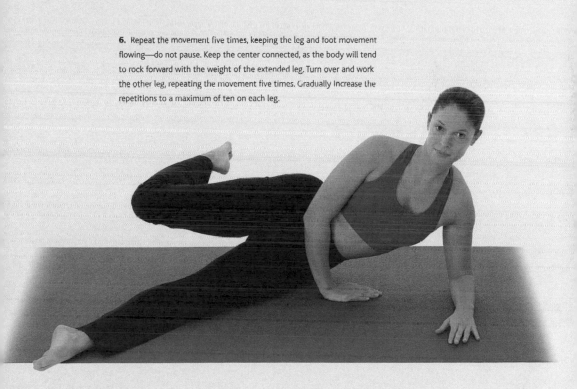

INNER THIGH LIFT

96

As you carry out this movement, do not just lift the leg up and down—really feel the inner thigh muscle working from the knee to the pubic bone, as if you were resisting gravity. As in the previous exercise, do not let the ribs sink or collapse to the floor. Keep the ribs connected to a strong center, so that your body is strong from the pelvis to the shoulder.

Aim: To stretch and strengthen the inner and outer thighs.
Benefits: The abdominals and the inner and outer thighs.

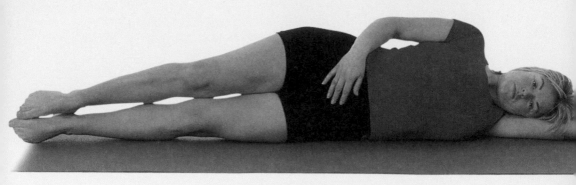

1. Lie on your side, with your hips stacked one on top of the other and your legs together with the inner thighs connected. Extend your lower arm, palm up, so that you are in a straight line from your fingertips to your toes. Keep your head in line with your spine, with your chin forward.

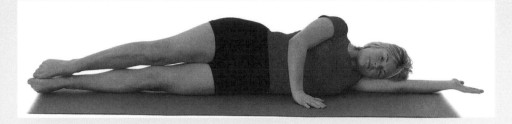

2. Inhale, and as you do so place the palm of your lower hand on the floor to aid in pressing you up.

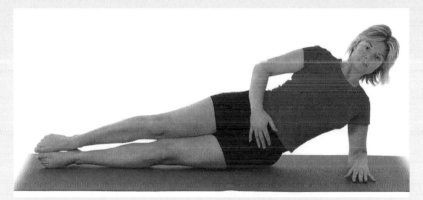

3. Exhale, and draw your lower arm in toward your body, placing the elbow directly under your shoulder and the forearm on its side, with the fingers pointed away from the body. Keep the top shoulder in neutral, and rest the palm of the upper hand across the navel for feedback.

4. Now angle your legs forwards slightly, without changing the position of your spine, which must still be in a straight line from your head to your tail.

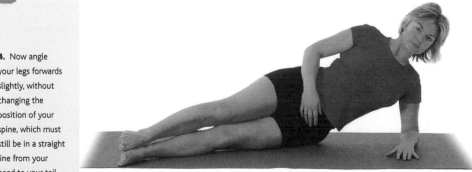

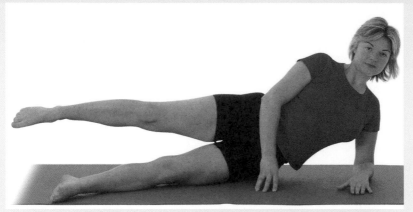

5. From this position, separate the top leg and bring it back in line with your hip joint.

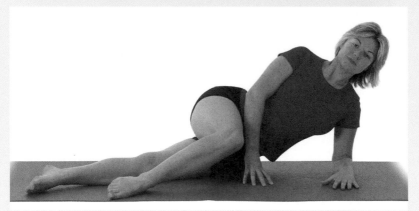

6. Bend the top leg at the knee into a figure 4.

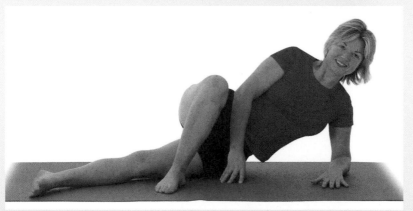

7. Then place the foot on the floor in front of the bottom leg, with the bottom leg fully extended.

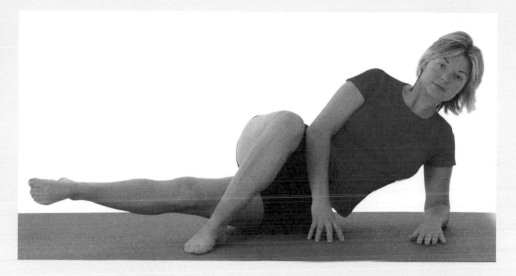

8. Inhale and lift up the bottom leg, keeping the leg straight but without locking the knee.

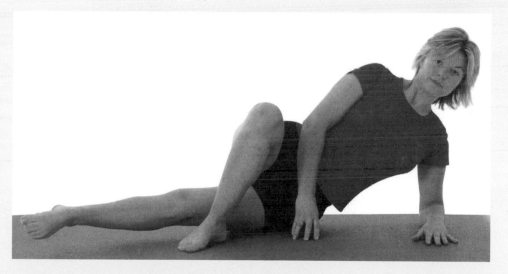

9. Exhale and lower the leg without touching the floor. Repeat the movement five times, without touching the floor between repetitions. Turn over and work the other leg, repeating the movement five times. Gradually increase the number of repetitions to a maximum of ten on each side.

BICEPS CURL

97

This exercise is for toning the upper arm to the front. The action is rather like raising the lower arm from a hinge at the elbow. For this exercise and the following one, you will need either small hand weights or two food cans of equal weight—baked beans, for example.

Aim: To work the muscle at the top of the upper arm, which flexes your arm toward your body.
Benefits: The biceps muscle.

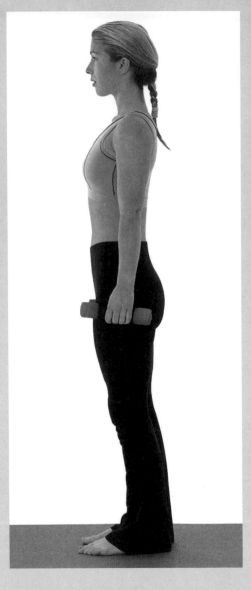

1. Stand with your knees slightly bent, but not locked, and your feet placed evenly under your hips. Hang your arms loosely by your sides, palms toward you. Relax your shoulders into neutral and make sure there is no tension in any part of the body.

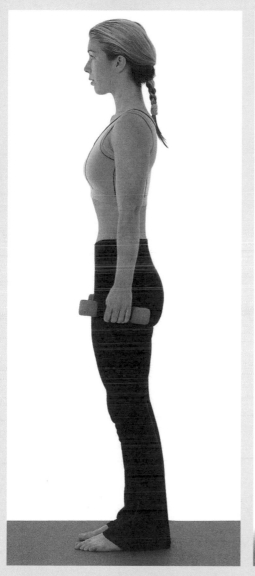

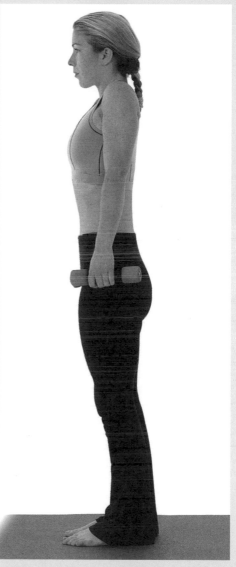

2. Inhale, then exhale to connect the center, gently drawing up on the pelvic floor and drawing the navel back to the spine.

3. Inhale and shrug your shoulders toward your ears, then exhale, feeling your shoulder blades melting down your back into neutral.

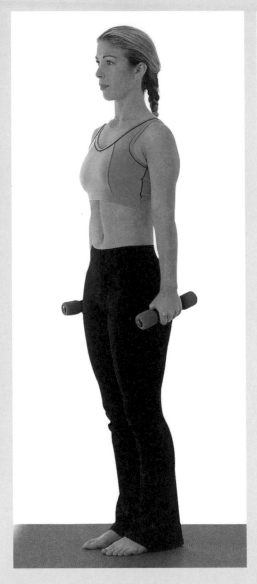

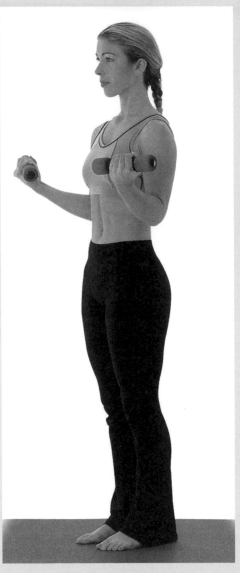

4. Inhale, keeping your arms full-length.

5. Exhale and start to curl your arms at the elbows toward your body. As the lower arms move upward, twist them so that the palms are now facing your body. At the top of the movement, your forearms will be facing your body with your palms just below the chin.

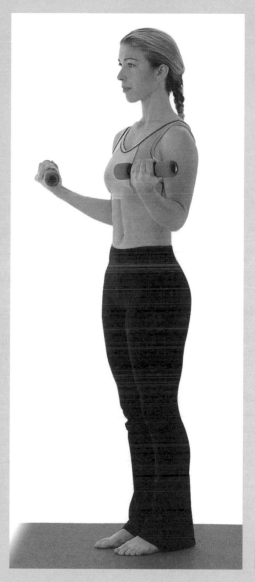

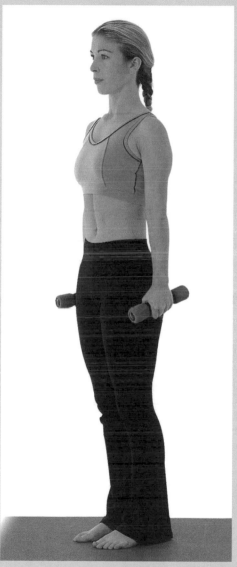

6. Inhale and lower the arms, twisting them so that the palms are facing your sides at the end of the movement.

7. Gradually repeat the movement to make a total of ten.

TRICEPS KICKBACKS

This exercise is for toning the triceps at the back of the upper arm, traditionally a slack muscle in women. Again, the elbow acts as a hinge to take the lower arm away from the body. It is essential that you keep the center connected while you are bending over, to protect the spine.

Aim: To work the muscle at the back of the upper arm, which extends the lower arm.
Benefits: The triceps muscle.

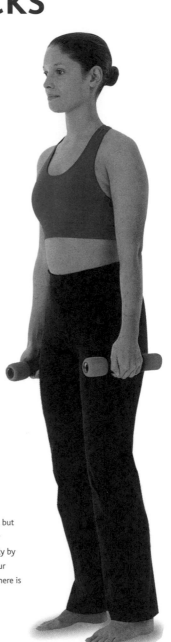

1. Stand with your knees slightly bent, but not locked, and your feet placed evenly under your hips. Hang your arms loosely by your sides, palms toward you. Relax your shoulders into neutral and make sure there is no tension in any part of the body.

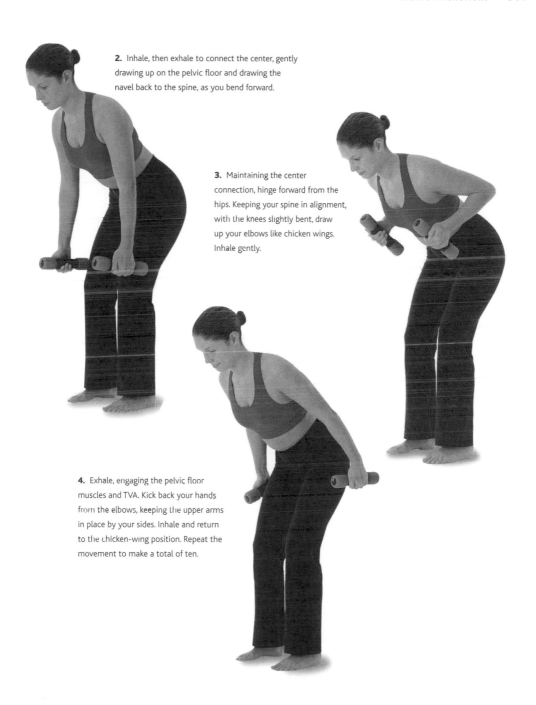

2. Inhale, then exhale to connect the center, gently drawing up on the pelvic floor and drawing the navel back to the spine, as you bend forward.

3. Maintaining the center connection, hinge forward from the hips. Keeping your spine in alignment, with the knees slightly bent, draw up your elbows like chicken wings. Inhale gently.

4. Exhale, engaging the pelvic floor muscles and TVA. Kick back your hands from the elbows, keeping the upper arms in place by your sides. Inhale and return to the chicken-wing position. Repeat the movement to make a total of ten.

ADVANCED ONE HUNDRED

99

This is the ultimate Pilates exercise, for which all earlier movements have prepared you. Your central stability must be 100 percent for this, so you will need all the core and lower abdominal strength gained from previous exercises such as Abdominals 1 and 2, Lower Abdominals, Lumbar Roll, and Knee Folds. You must have the pelvis in neutral when performing this exercise, and the shoulder girdle set, and your back must not be flattened or arched out of its natural curves.

1. Lie on your back, with your knees at 45 degrees and your feet in line with your knees. Rest your arms by your sides, palms down. Inhale, lengthening through the body and feeling relaxed. Exhale, connecting the pelvic floor and drawing the navel back to the spine. Inhale.

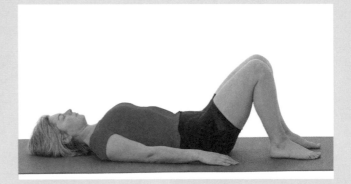

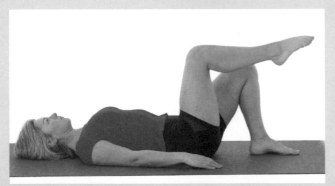

2. Exhale, maintaining the connection with the center, and raise the right leg to 90 degrees. Inhale, maintaining the connection with the leg at 90 degrees.

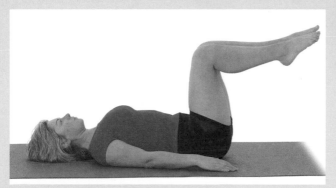

3. Exhale, reinforce the connection with the center, and raise the left leg to 90 degrees, alongside the right leg. Inhale.

4. Exhale, flexing the upper body forward with the arms extended from the shoulders and hovering above the floor. Keep the shoulder girdle in neutral with no tension. Both upper and lower body are now flexed toward the center.

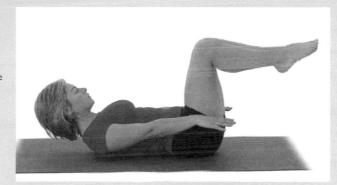

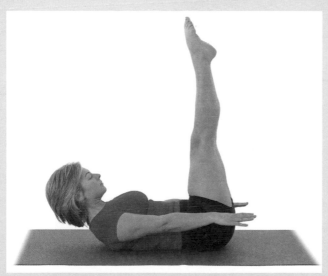

5. Fully extend the legs toward the ceiling. Inhale for a count of five and maintain the position—do not let the upper body release back to the floor. Exhale for a count of five, maintaining the connection to the center. Maintain the position as you continue to breathe, inhaling for a count of five and exhaling for a count of five each time. Aim to repeat the exercise ten times, without losing form—ten repetitions by ten breaths makes the Pilates Advanced One Hundred.

SINGLE LEG STRETCH WITH OBLIQUES

Aim: To stabilize the pelvis, strengthen the obliques and lower abdominals, and mobilize the hips.
Benefits: Transversus abdominis, hip flexors/extensors, and obliques.

As with the Advanced One Hundred (*see* pages 310–311), you must have the pelvis in neutral when performing this exercise, and the shoulder girdle set, and your back must not be flattened or arched out of its natural curves. Good stability at the center is essential as you are aiming for a controlled, deliberate twist using the oblique muscles, without rocking from side to side. Keep your elbows open as you perform the move, and do not be tempted to bring them in toward your head.

1. Lie on your back, with your knees at 45 degrees and your feet in line with your knees. Rest your arms by your sides, palms down. Inhale, lengthening through the body and feeling relaxed. Exhale, connecting the pelvic floor and drawing the navel back to the spine. Inhale.

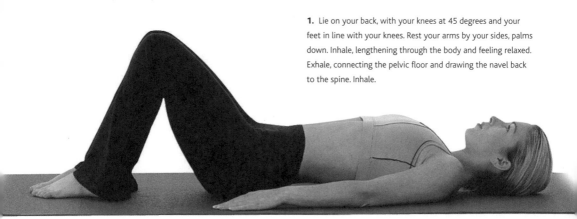

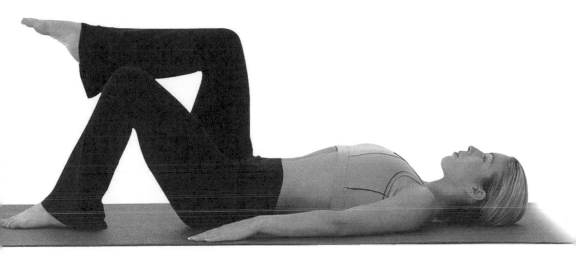

2. Exhale and allow one knee to float slowly up toward the ceiling, as if being pulled by an invisible string. Stop when the knee is in line with the hip and the angle of the knee is 90 degrees. Inhale, maintaining 30 percent TVA activation and keeping the leg bent at 90 degrees. Exhale, reinforce the connection with the center and raise the other knee to 90 degrees. Inhale.

3. Exhale, flexing the upper body forward with the arms extended from the shoulders and hovering above the floor. Keep the shoulder girdle in neutral with no tension. Both upper and lower body are now flexed toward the center.

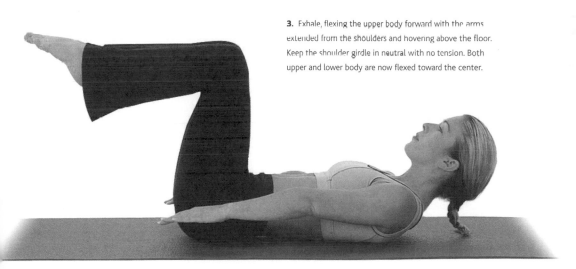

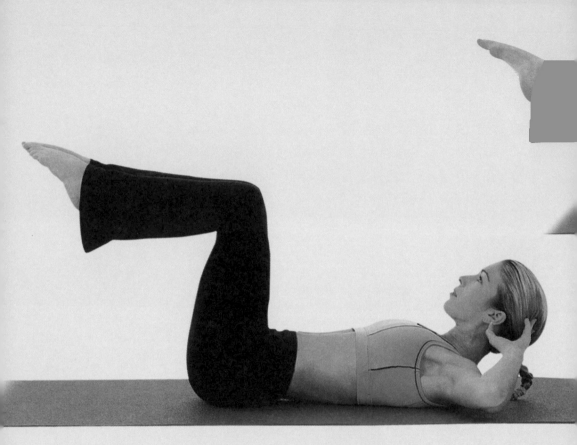

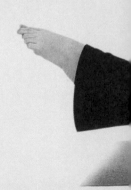

4. Bring your hands to the sides of your head but keep your elbows open. Inhale, to prepare.

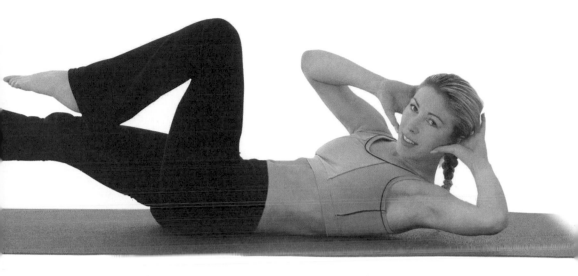

5. Exhale, extend your right leg away from the center, and twist at the waist to take your right shoulder to the left knee.

6. Inhale and return body and leg to the center. Exhale, extend your left leg away from the center, and twist at the waist to take your left shoulder to the right knee. Repeat the exercise five times, gradually increasing to a maximum of ten.

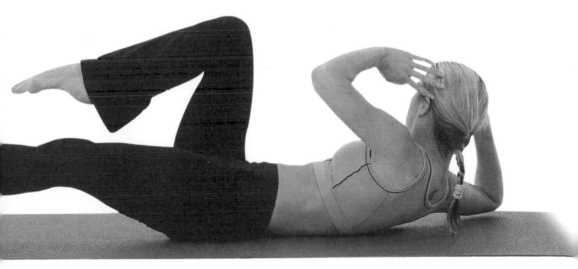

GLOSSARY TO PILATES

ABDOMINAL HOLLOWING
Engaging the abdominal muscles so that the abdomen can support and maintain easy, flowing movement.

ABDOMINALS
The muscles around the spine in the lower back that initiate movement and support and maintain good posture.

ALIGNMENT
Balancing the body so that the weight is distributed evenly over both feet and the skeleton maintains its natural alignment.

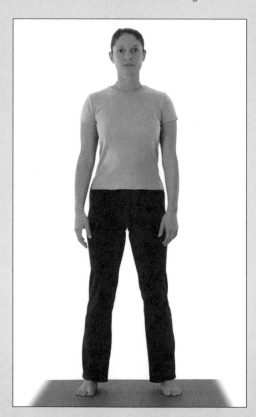

BREATHING
Correct breathing is essential in Pilates, and it is very important to follow the inhale/exhale instructions.

BUCKET HANDLE
The Pilates breath expands the diaphragm and pushes out the ribcage, like a bucket handle being lifted up and out.

CENTER
The area around the middle of the body, which must be strong and stable to initiate flowing movement.

CERVICAL SPINE
The bones at the top of the spine where it joins the head, more usually referred to as the neck.

CONTROL
Controlled movements are essential in Pilates, to ensure that each movement is flowing and graceful.

CORE
Another name for the center of the body, from which good posture and all movement stems.

CORE CONDITIONING
Working on the muscles at the center or core of the body to promote optimum strength and stability.

DORSIFLEX
To flex the foot at the ankle so that the toes point forward and the back of the leg is stretched.

FEEDBACK
The exchange of information between mind and body that takes place during exercise, to ensure that movements are correctly carried out.

Left: Always make sure that your weight is distributed evenly over both feet.

FLOWING MOVEMENT

Taking one movement into the next in a natural, flowing way, without any hesitation or jerky action.

GAZE

In Pilates, it is important to keep your gaze on the horizon to help maintain a good body position.

GIRDLE OF STRENGTH

The name used to describe the center or core of the body, which the Pilates technique aims to strengthen and stabilize, to promote flowing movement and good posture.

LUMBAR MULTIFIDUS

One of the muscles in the center that works with the transversus abdominis, to promote easy movement and good posture.

MODIFICATION

A suggestion for changing a move to make it a little easier until full strength and stability have been achieved in the center.

MOTIVATION

Keeping in mind the reason for practicing Pilates, for example, to overcome physical ailments or to promote a feeling of well-being.

NEUTRAL

In Pilates, this means relaxing the shoulder girdle, spine, and pelvis into their natural positions, so that they are not forced or tilted either to left or right, or forward or backward.

PELVIS PLANTARFLEX

The bones supporting the torso at the base, to which the spine and legs are attached. The pelvic floor muscles support the abdominal muscles to promote movement.

POSTURE

The position in which the body is held. Poor posture can lead to a variety of ailments, and Pilates aims to eliminate this by improving posture.

PRECISION

It is important to carry out Pilates movements with precision—that is, exactly as they are described in the step-by-step instructions.

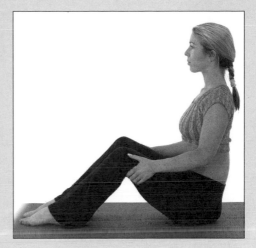

Above: It is important to keep your gaze on the horizon.

PLANTARFLEX

To stretch the foot at the ankle so that the toes point straight out, in alignment with the leg.

PROGRESSION

A suggestion for changing a move to make it more difficult once full strength and stability have been achieved in the center.

SHOULDER GIRDLE

The group of bones that make up the shoulders, including the shoulder blades, collarbones, and upper arm bones.

SPINE

The column of bones running from the base of the head to the tail of the torso, which connects and supports the skeletal system.

TRANSVERSUS ABDOMINIS

The deep postural muscle found in the center of the body, which is key to promoting flowing movement and good posture.

VISUALIZATION

Creating and maintaining a clear picture of the desired outcome of any activity.

INDEX